A PEACEFUL GUT, MIND & BODY

Finding a new you through your gut

Dr Angela Genoni

A peaceful gut, mind & body

Cover illustration and in text pillar image, created with the use of Canva Pro AI

ISBN: 978-1-923512-14-6 (Paperback)

NATIONAL LIBRARY OF AUSTRALIA

A catalogue record for this book is available from the National Library of Australia

Self-Published by Angela Genoni with assistance by Clark & Mackay
Proudly printed in Australia by Clark & Mackay

CONTENTS

FOREWORD

I studied nutrition back in the early 2000s at University, in the days when obesity was considered purely a calorie excess problem. The solution was, at the time, to restrict calories without much thought to how that restriction impacted the way people perceived their bodies.

Yes, to lose weight we absolutely need to reduce our food intake, but I think we messed it all up in the process. We turned a basic human need with emotions and feelings attached to it into a maths problem. We forgot to help people understand how their body actually works. To give them the love and appreciation for themselves and what their body CAN do instead of what it can't.

We focused on restriction to achieve perfection, and now we have a generation of folks who think badly of themselves every time they look in the mirror. We can't see the wonder in those legs that helped us hike up that mountain last year, the amazement of that stomach that once held babies inside it, or the sun freckles from that relaxing holiday a few weeks ago. We just forgot to stop, appreciate and respect our own bodies.

As a young nutritionist, I was just like everyone else with my views on eating and diets. However, my views started to change when I did my PhD looking at the impact of longer-term diets on the gut microbiome. I saw some (actually a lot of) people who were really picky about what they ate, to the point where they wouldn't eat out with friends. At the time I only briefly wondered about the healthiness of this "perfection" but in hindsight, it left a lasting impact on me. After my PhD, I worked for a nonprofit organisation that also promoted a very strict diet. Again, the big picture message was always lost in arguing over the fine details. There is more to a diet than just food. It is comfort, it is time with friends, it is relaxation. Whatever it is to you, it is always more than just the actual food. This is also what makes it so tricky when we try to be sensible.

People get very feisty when it comes to "diets"…

We all eat, we all know how food impacts us, so we all have a valid opinion. Social media is full of these opinions. It worked for them (or it appeared to), so it must work for everyone, right? Unfortunately, although our human bodies are super similar, they are also very different at the same time. So, what worked for that influencer might not work for you. Can you prepare the same meals each week as they do? Do you have the same work schedule? Do they have kids to drive around all afternoon like you? There are so many areas where food needs to fit into our lives that it is near on impossible to follow a meal plan or some strict diet without causing you some level of guilt as early as day two or three.

It's your diet, your life, no one else's.

We just need to help you design your food around your life and make it work for you.

I've spent many years studying the complex science of the gut microbiome. I can tell some wonderous things about some of the biochemical pathways that happen in the gut, how we extract bacterial DNA from poop samples and all of the complexities around food, food matrices and food processing. But as I am now older and wiser, I really feel the value for most people is being able to understand all this complex science in a way that is applicable to real life. So, I've taken my Aussie humour, my complex science and my love of being kind and compassionate and put it all together to paint you the big picture, because at the end of the day, that's what really matters. I'm always up for a chat about a scientific paper and perhaps the limitations of the statistics they used, but really, I'm most interested in what that paper means for you and your lifestyle.

This book will give you the guidance to help you appreciate your body for the wonderous things it does for you, to help you understand the power of those little bacterial friends living in your gut and to guide you with small and sustainable changes to get rid of any guilt you might have about going on "another diet". You literally can't fail when you set yourself up for success by starting small.

It is a good idea to digest (throwing puns in already) all of the information here first, then head to the plan in the self-assessment section, where you actually map out the things that are important to you and your plan for getting yourself there.

This journey then is about a shift in perspective and stacking some small changes together, which might in isolation, seem insignificant, but when combined over two to three months, is suddenly enough to transform your whole life.

In keeping with my views that diets are much more than food, we also delve into the things that can also significantly influence our gut and overall health, such as things like exercise, time in nature and time with friends. Things that those influencers trying to sell you that supplement seem to forget.

Let's start a new generation of people who love and respect their bodies and as a result, find it easy to nurture themselves.

CHAPTER 1

Mirror Mirror on the Wall

You've picked up this book for a reason, right?

You might be having some gut issues. Or maybe you are just sick of feeling confused because you are just not sure what is going on with that bloating? Or you're sick of dieting and trying completely wacky and unsustainable things?

In case you haven't already guessed, I absolutely love what I do. The more I talk to people about the need to shift perspective and focus on the positive and learn about the gut, the more determined I am to talk to more people!

I genuinely want to help you love, respect and nurture your body. And this starts with knowing it a little better. So, some of this book might seem a little bit like high school human biology, but as adults who eat a lot of food every day, this information is kind of important, so as you read this bit, try and appreciate the wonder of it all.

The details of digestion are hugely complex and I still stop and say "wow" often when I delve into new things about how specialised some of our cells are and how they behave in certain circumstances. Although we know much about the human body, there is also much still to learn. This is a part of why I take the food approach and generally don't recommend supplements (we will get into this later).

Knowing your body a little better is one step, but before we start on this, I want you to think about what you said to yourself the last time you looked in the mirror.

Was it: "oh man, I really need to start dieting again, I'm outta control right now", or "I hate my thighs being so fat" or "why aren't the scales down today, I'm so crap at diets"

OR

"I'm so grateful these arms are strong enough to carry my toddler around all day", or "these legs mean I can walk to work and save the train/fuel money today", or "this tummy had a baby in it only a few months/years ago. Wow"

Think about the feeling you get when you read the first lot of thoughts vs the second.

There is a massive difference in the effect on your mood and the rest of your day from just this one self-narrative. The second celebrates yourself; it encourages you to be kinder to yourself because damn, you are amazing. Whereas the first one almost always puts you in a bad mood before you even get out the door for the morning.

So, what are three things you are grateful that your body CAN do or has done recently?

Write these down and put them on your bathroom mirror or anywhere where you talk down to yourself. You might need to say them repeatedly (saying them out loud is even better) for a few weeks, but slowly and surely, the benefits will start to sink into your subconscious. Then before you know it, you might start thinking, wow… I carried a 20kg two-year-old all day yesterday. How awesome am I?

Sometimes these self-defeating thoughts came from somewhere; they came from someone in our past telling us we were fat, we weren't loved if we didn't fit into that dress or we just didn't get appreciated or loved enough for who we were inside at the time. If you are finding you are replaying these scenarios or memories out in your head too much, it might be worth reminding yourself that most of the time, these comments reflect insecurity in the person saying them. They come from a place where they don't know about nutrition, about how the body works, or about how much more wholesome life is when we don't focus on the superficial. It is almost always saying more about them than it is about you.

You can find your confidence again, and it starts with loving your body properly so that the desire to nurture it comes back.

CHAPTER 2

We Got Diets all Wrong

I'm writing this book around the wrong way on purpose. If you've picked up the book because you've been suffering from gut issues, then thinking about these next two chapters BEFORE you focus on your diet, will put you in a much better place to be successful, than focusing on diet alone.

Science tells us that diet is the biggest contributor to gut microbiome composition, but lifestyle and environment are important too, and in fact psychologically, I think they can make or break your diet and overall gut success.

If your mindset is not right or you're doing a diet with anxiety about everything you are eating, then it makes sense that it might not have much impact in terms of fixing your gut. The gut-brain axis knows you're still stressed about everything and keeps things in this stressed-out state of having a difficult gut.

You already know when your gut reacts to stressful situations; this is the gut and the brain talking to one another. So, if we do all this great work on our diet, but are still stressed out, or even worse, we get so anxious about what we are eating, then, of course, it cancels the benefits of the better diet out anyway. Compared to neighbouring residents with similar diets, Tibetan monks who practise deep meditation, have much greater gut microbiome diversity (a good thing) and lower cholesterol levels (1). Although this was only a small study, it highlights the sheer power of our mind and the control it can have over our total health journey.

Over the past year, I've read a lot of books on the power of thinking, and many of these have been quite transformative for me personally. Although I never started reading these for any gut reason, they've certainly highlighted the power of something science does not fully understand yet.

Challenging your thinking about your thinking might just be one of the most powerful things you do during or after this book. The way you talk to yourself matters.

The way you think about food matters.

The way you think about nourishing yourself matters.

Coming from a place of restricting yourself or feeling guilt for anything food-related is never going to be successful in the long term.

The great dieting experiment of the last couple of decades has been a complete flop. We know that at least one-third of people who went on any sort of diet regained most of the weight they lost within plus more within 5 years of stopping their diet (2). Aside from the health risks of regaining the weight you lost, it doesn't make you feel good, when you did all that work but didn't or weren't able to maintain it, does it?

There are several problems with the way we've done diets in the last two decades:

1. We tell people they aren't good enough as they are and base their progress on superficial outcomes.
2. The restriction that comes with any sort of diet or meal plan, has a very negative impact on our mindset and self-talk.
3. We haven't helped people understand the why behind it all so that they can care about their bodies on the inside.
4. We make too many changes with clients all at once, which is unsustainable once the initial motivation wears off. For some of us, we can sustain the motivation until we've lost a good amount of weight, for others, this might only last a week or two.

Telling yourself you can't eat something because you're dieting, places your mindset squarely in the case of restriction, deprivation or missing out. You might be dieting to lose weight, which further compounds this, because we're only focused on the superficial goal of looking a certain way. So, when we look in the mirror, all we have in our mind are the negative thoughts about how much more we need to lose, how unhappy we are with our body right now or how much do we need to restrict ourselves today, it's mostly negative and completely unhelpful for the long term. Because when we can't stick with this type of unrealistic plan, we get further down on ourselves.

See the negative cycle here?

If you want to break free of the diet industry and actually focus on getting properly healthy, we've got to work on the mindset stuff first. The diet is kind of secondary.

Have a think about why you chose this book. Are you struggling with a gut issue? Are you sick of dieting and saw this might offer something different? Or was it some other reason?

What is your major goal for your health for the next 12 months? Your goal should not have ANYTHING to do with how you look. Focus in on something incredibly positive and empowering, so that when you achieve it, you can look back and go "wow, I am smashing it", this was the year for me!

Your goal might be to learn to run 5km and do it without stopping,

To be able to walk up the stairs at work without puffing,

To get fit enough to go hiking in Peru,

To get strong enough to lift x kg at the gym,

To get strong enough to do a pull-up,

You get the idea here. Do you see how much more positive this is than telling yourself you have to lose something?

If you have a goal and you really want to achieve it, and it is such a positive thing for your life, there is a much better chance you'll get to achieving it – AND sustaining it, than if you wrote something like, "I want to lose 10kg".

So, write down your goal/s that you want to achieve for your health for the coming year. Make them achievable but massively positive.

Having positive goals instead of restrictive or negative ones is also a lot more fun. Diets are more than food, so let's remember that. Some of the longest-living cultures on earth, yes, they have awesome diets, but they also live very traditionally in terms of their family and social structures. They prepare food together, they eat together and some partake in afternoon siestas (3,4). Research often hones in on the diet aspect, but we really can't overlook the reduction in stress that comes from this type of lifestyle.

Western societies are very individualist, we are focused on achieving things for ourselves, and our success is often judged as such. This actually places a lot of stress on us because not only do we feel like we have to achieve things and be kicking goals all the time for our work/career, but we are also expected to cook five-star meals and work out, all while juggling running a house. Sound familiar?

We can't change the society in which we live super easily, (I am trying here, ok?!), but we can change the way we think about it. We can change how we manage it. Being aware of these pressures and knowing they are real, that they are valid, and that they often get in the way of healthy lifestyles is the most important and biggest first step to managing them better in your own household.

Now the next step on this journey is getting you there. We need to give you the confidence to step off the diet wagon and learn to listen to your body again. The goal is to get enough balance back to feel at peace with the why behind what we want to achieve and be confident with our strategy to get there.

CHAPTER 3

The FOUR Pillars of Gut Health

Gut health is really referring to having a happy population of gut bacteria in your colon. But to get to this point, it is much, much more complicated than just taking a supplement or going on a diet. Yes, diet is one of the biggest drivers of microbiome composition (5,6), but the big picture involves other aspects too, which is why I created a four-pillared approach. All of the four pillars are underpinned by our mindset. The knowledge and application is great, but the mindset is the most important.

Before we delve into the four pillars, I want to re-emphasise the importance of reflecting on how we think. How do you talk to yourself? How do you think about your body? How do you think about the things your body does? How much do you currently stop and appreciate the hard work your body does on the inside?

While you ponder these questions, I'll explain the concept of breaking down true gut health (which will flow on to your overall health) into the pillars. The chapters after this cover all these pillars (just not in the same order), plus there's some practical information on how to apply all of this knowledge into your lifestyle, how to structure your time and some reframing of your thinking about your priorities. As you read on, think about how ALL of these things are important for not only your gut health, but also your overall health.

PILLAR ONE: BACTERIAL FUEL

Fibre and gut bacterial composition. One of the biggest factors to influence our bacterial friends. This area is, however, not as simplistic as it might sound. There are so many different types of fibre and foods which have the ability to shift our gut populations. Upskilling yourself on the workings of the gut and all the nuances with food and fibres will totally put you ahead of the game here.

PILLAR TWO: BACTERIAL "SUPPLEMENTS"

Other food components that shift bacterial abundances. There are many other things in the food we eat. Things such as polyphenols for example, the colourful parts of fruits and vegetables, do not fall under the definition of fibre, but can still provide a big impact in terms of changing what the populations of bacteria in our colon can do (similar to vitamins for humans. The bacteria don't use them for energy, but they still rely on them). Similarly, ultra-processed foods, with their additives and preservatives, can also give things a shake-up on the inside and it is important to acknowledge this as we start to make some small changes.

PILLAR THREE: HOW WE LIVE

Lifestyle factors. It is pretty amazing to think that something like exercise can shift and change the populations of bacteria in our colon. So, if you're struggling with your gut right now, having a bit of an understanding of the "why" behind some of the gut tips can really put you back on top in terms of managing your symptoms. This pillar also explores things like alcohol and stress management, which are super important for managing not only your gut health but your overall happiness too.

PILLAR FOUR: SOCIAL AND ENVIRONMENTAL

Your environment can contribute to your gut health too. We will talk some more in later chapters about getting outside and how being social might benefit more than just our peace and happiness.

I'm sure you already noticed if you've been on a diet before, that while it might provide you some guidance on how to eat, it doesn't help you understand the why behind the diet, nor incorporate the other factors to ensure that you can actually create a healthy and complete lifestyle for yourself. Putting all the pieces together is really the key.

The pillars of gut health are like trees in our garden. They won't grow unless the soil is right (our mindset) or if we don't water them (with our knowledge and understanding of the big picture).

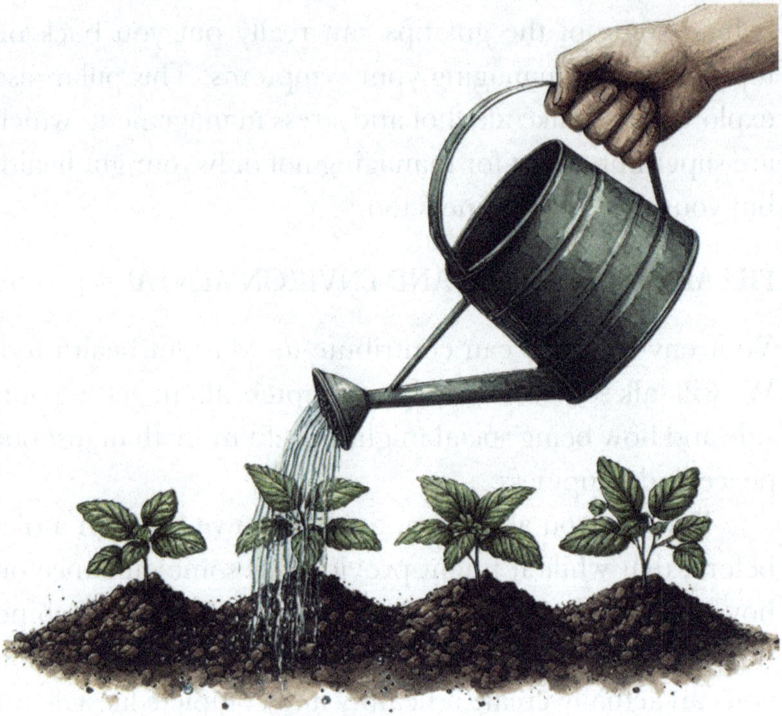

MINDSET

CHAPTER 4

Choose Yourself

THE QUALITY OF THE SOIL MATTERS

If you feel like your health has held you back lately, let's say it might have made you 20% less productive over the last 5 years; then financially, there has been a big cost to you personally, for not nurturing yourself. I'm not pointing this out because I want you to dwell on it; in fact, it is quite the opposite. You are here because you want to do something different. Most of society is perfectly happy operating at a reduced level of productivity.

So, there is now a huge opportunity for you because you want to grow and learn and be the best version of yourself. There is great value well beyond just feeling better and having a better, more comfortable gut, you can quite literally, be ahead of the game in terms of other achievements too.

What is your why?

Visualise yourself six months from now, having achieved all your health goals. What will that give you? Will that mean you've got more energy to spend play time with your kids? To be more productive at work and achieve your career goals? Focusing on not just the end goal, but also WHY you want this, makes it more likely to become your reality.

I want you to write down somewhere, to remind yourself: What are your three biggest reasons for coming on this journey? They can't be physical things. They need to describe how you want to feel at the end of this journey. Write these down like you already have them. Put them somewhere you can see them. Look at them and say them to yourself as often as you need to. Daily is a good idea.

For example, I no longer stress about what I am eating, and I am relaxed enough to invest that energy in spending quality time with my partner/kids.

I nurture my body with good food, exercise and time with friends and family.

"***The time you spend investing in yourself is one of the BEST investments you will ever make***"

When I always ask my clients to put themselves on the top of the priority list for the week. I'm almost always met with "I've got kids, or got work etc".

What sort of parent, carer, or partner to do really want to be? Who do you aspire to be and show up as in your life? Make yourself a mind map on a piece of paper and write it down. Who are you and what do you stand for? Put a "who am I" in the centre and lines to all the things that are part of who you want to be. For example, mine had "I am kind and empathetic towards others", "I am a present parent when I am with the kids" and "I exercise because of the way it makes me feel, during and afterwards". If you write them in the present tense, even if you don't think you actually do those things yet, it shifts your mindset into a state of moving towards that person.

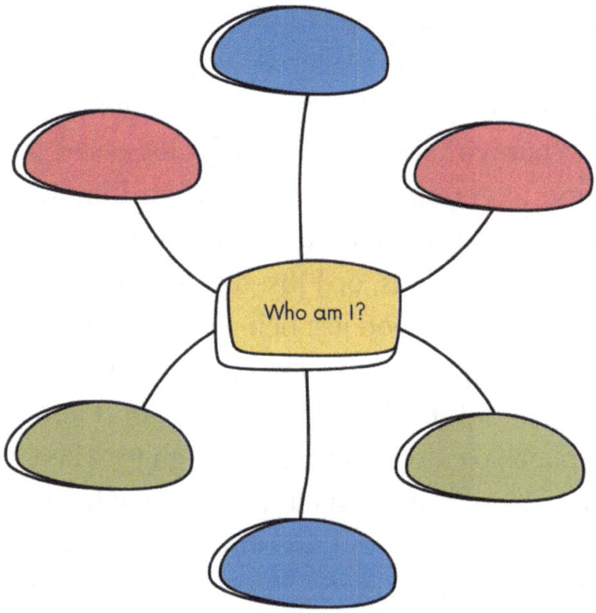

Doing this exercise for me really shifted my thinking and my self-confidence all at once. It highlighted to me how important it was for me to show up to my kids as caring, present, relaxed and kind. I know I can be all of those things and more if I'm feeling good. And feeling good for me is feeling fit and having enough sleep.

It's hard to show up for anyone when we feel like crap, let alone ourselves. That is why YOU need to be at the top of your list.

"*No one is going to show up for you, except you*".

So, what are the top couple of things that are at the absolute top of your list? What do you need to do with your health to support this and bring it to fruition?

It certainly makes it a heck of a lot easier to find the motivation to get out for exercise, when I know I feel like I'm living up to my full potential afterwards, when I have a fun day with the kids, or I just feel happy because of it.

You get to feel good just being you, and that means it's easier to show up for all your other responsibilities.

It's all about making a plan A, a plan B and a plan C. Making plans so extreme that you feel guilty when you don't meet them doesn't work. Making a plan that has enough flex and give to work with the pressures of life when the week turns upside down is key. So, if you make a plan A, great, make it achievable. Make a plan B, for what you'll do if you don't feel up to the plan A. And plan C, for when all things are upside down, what can you still achieve?

I need to point out, that this is not about giving yourself an out. This is purely about being realistic. As humans, we tend to make harsh rules for ourselves like "I'm going to go to the gym EVERY DAY!". This is a really nice idea, but let's face it, who actually does that? So, the plans are not to give you an excuse, they are to encourage you to think about what is actually possible, rather than a pie-in-the-sky type goal that sets you up for failure.

Let's map it out with a fitness example as it is an easy one to overestimate!

From the mind map: I keep fit because I enjoy being active with the kids, it is great time together.

Plan A: Feeling fit to me is being able to run, 4 times per week.

Plan B: If work gets busy, I can still fit in a 30-minute slow and easy run before the kids get up. It's only 30 minutes. OR I can shuffle my days exercise days around depending on work commitments.

Plan C: If the kids are all sick (or I'm not feeling the best), I can still get outside for a walk. OR I can at least do two or three sessions each week.

I want to give you a reminder that this is an ongoing challenge and not necessarily something that comes naturally. I'm living the challenges with you. I've got three teenagers, taken on too much work, got a house, kids sport etc. I get it. But putting yourself at the top of that list is something that you need to do consciously each and every week. Show up for yourself, **especially** when you don't want to. *Being consistent gets results.* Showing up even when you didn't want to, is so empowering! My absolute best exercise sessions always seem to happen on the days I really had to drag myself out of bed. Maybe I just had no expectation that it was going to be a good session, I don't know. All I know is that the hardest part is just getting out the door. The rest is actually easy. And often once you're out the door, good things might just happen. It doesn't matter if it is a simple ten-minute walk or a two-hour run, getting out the door is the key bit.

You don't need to make massive changes to be better at anything. Small changes are doable and more achievable.

So, choose to show up for yourself each and every day, even in the smallest way possible.

CHAPTER 5

The Joy of Simple Changes

KEEPING THE PERSPECTIVE WITH YOUR KNOWLEDGE

As a young nutritionist I grew up watching shows like Biggest Loser, where the poor contestants were ridiculed in their own homes for whatever was in their fridge and pantry. Yes, they needed to make some changes, but think about how you would feel if your whole routine of buying, making and preparing food got thrown on its head. As I've become older (and wiser, according to my grey hair) it has really become apparent that this is totally NOT the right way to make lasting change. No wonder most people put back on the weight they lost plus some extra, when they go on extreme diets. It's easy to maintain some motivation for short periods (for some people), but when $hit gets busy on Wednesday after you had an awful meeting at work and you had to drive the kids around all afternoon, what do you do? You fall back on the routines and habits that you took a lifetime to develop. You pick up pizza on the way home. I don't blame you. Our constant busy-ness is always exhausting us, our society just has not valued the joy of eating simple meals prepared at home. It's the constant commercialisation of food marketed as quick and easy.

This is why, when we want to make actual lasting change, we have to set ourselves up to succeed, so we literally can't fail. My number one piece of advice from this whole book, is to only make one small change at a time. The smaller the better. Make a tiny change, and wait till it is embedded in your routine, before you add on the next one. This way we can put a gold star on our own chart on the fridge at the end of the week, and then we can feel like we are achieving and winning. Play the little mind game with yourself and watch your confidence roll in.

Most people (in Australia, it is around 95% (7)) don't eat the recommended servings of fruits and vegetables. So, this is always an easy place to start. We want to keep the focus on adding something positive, without any restriction or anything negative. There is no guilt anywhere to be seen when you work with me. By default, if you add some more fruits and vegetables, at some point this will detract you from eating some of the less desirable foods that have perhaps become regulars in your diet, but you don't really need to concentrate on this for now. Let's get some extra fruits and vegetables in first before we focus on anything extra.

Make it as simple as you possibly can so you can't fail it. It might be packing a simple raw carrot from the pack in the fridge in your lunchbox or taking an apple a day.

Whatever fruit or vegetable you decide, you need to make some plans for how you are going to do this.

People tend to dismiss this bit because it seems well, quite silly, but what are you going to do if you run out of carrots? You're only giving yourself such a simple task, so make sure you plan what you do if the day turns pear-shaped (pardon the pun). If there's a supermarket near work, then you can go buy some at lunch. And if you get swayed by any of the fast snack items at the checkout. Don't beat yourself up, just eat your fruit or veg FIRST.

The more we crowd out some of the less healthy things in our diet with the better things, the less we even have to think about it. Remember it is the shift in your perspective too, which can literally transform your life. So don't focus on negatives or restrictions, focus on the things you CAN do and the things you CAN add. Make a mental note of how grateful you are that you GET to make these changes in your life.

Once you've got this first amendment to your diet nailed, then you can move on to the next one. It's stacking small changes on top of each other, and then before we know it, our whole diet looks like an Instagram post.

I should also point out that our gut bacteria are very well adapted to different food sources. They've been used to being kept on their toes, so to speak, for thousands of years. Food might have been abundant one minute and scarce the next, but our bacteria are well-equipped to handle this change. We know that by drastically changing your diet, the gut bacteria shift also shapeshifts in as little as five days

(8). However, and there is a big caveat on however here, because this amount of change in a short period of time is going to be mighty uncomfortable. You'll spend most of your workday on the toilet or being bloated or gassy or all of the above. Not pleasant. The joy here is taking it slow. Give your little friends in your gut a bit of time to get on board with the extra fibre. Keeping your symptoms to a minimum. We want the diet change to be sustainable, remember, and it is well and truly more sustainable if we do it slowly and it doesn't kill us with stomach cramps in the meantime.

If you focus on just adding extra fruit and vegetables for a few weeks, just one each week until these are part of your daily routine, you will pretty quickly get to the point where you are eating the required serves, which is pretty cool.

Now, we've all got things we know we can work on, so at least for the first few weeks, adding things in is going to be super easy. The things you add don't need to be part of your meals either, they can be side things or snacks, which makes it even easier. Once we get past this part, you might need some guidance to help you work out which types of fibres are best for your gut and how to structure your meals to maximise your intake. I'll always have some good (and free) tips on my social media profiles, but just make sure the advice you get here is credible and remember you don't need to get sucked into buying anything extra in terms of superfoods or supplements unless medically necessary.

After the first few weeks, make sure you stop and take some time to reflect on how you are feeling. How have you been sleeping? How are your stress levels? Sometimes we are so busy we don't even take the time to stop and check in with ourselves about how we are feeling. Adding in a few extra serves of fruits and vegetables over a couple of weeks will be doing fantastic things for you on the inside, and I won't be at all surprised to hear that you realised you have been sleeping better, feeling less groggy in the mornings and have more energy during the work day.

As you go through the rest of the book, you'll also notice we talk a lot about non-food things that can also impact the gut. You should also implement these at the same pace and start small, just like our food modifications. You might like to include some changes over a month or so which have nothing to do with food, but are more around exercise or stress management. Make sure you celebrate these with as much joy as any food related change, because they are just as positive.

CHAPTER 6

Gut Health is Big Business

KEEPING THE PERSPECTIVE WITH YOUR KNOWLEDGE

The gut health industry is big business. When I started my PhD, there wasn't a lot of research on the gut microbiome, and more than a few people thought I had rocks in my head to examine poo for my thesis. [Side note: I was also skeptical about it, but having three small children at the time, did somewhat desensitise me to bodily excrements]

With the explosion in gut research also comes the commercialisation opportunities for all the different things that are studied. Fruit extracts used in a 4-week study suddenly hit the shelves with all sorts of health claims on them. I'm certainly not against some of these supplements, but the sheer quantity of them and the promotion of them relentlessly on our social media feeds, only gives us two things. First, it gives us the feeling we aren't good enough as we are. Second, it just adds to the overwhelm and confusion because how the heck are we supposed to decipher all the products, supplements and research to work out which of these might actually work and which ones are just snake oil?

My approach is to just keep it simple. Clear your mind that you "need" ANYTHING extra. You can get all the nutrition you need from food. That totally goes against the commercialisation of nutrition out there, but scientifically, it is 100% correct. I will say it again. You can meet all of your nutrition needs from food. Wow. You don't need to feel like you have to buy anything extra ever again. This is so freeing. Can you feel the weight lifting off your shoulders about now?

It is also a heck of a lot less expensive than all the stuff you probably already have in the cupboard. And I know from my past purchasing habits, that many of those supplements were tried for a couple of weeks, and then took up residence at the back of the cupboard to collect dust... Am I resonating here?

There is definitely a time and a place for supplements, but these should come with professional advice. For example, you might need a B12 supplement if you want to be completely plant-based, or you might need a targeted fibre supplement for specific IBS issues.

Now we have that clear, let's get onto gut health. Everyone talks about it, but not many people explain what it means, where the action happens and how we can change it.

CHAPTER 7

Everything Works Together

KEEPING THE PERSPECTIVE WITH YOUR KNOWLEDGE, THE PLANTS ALL GROW TOGETHER

The gut environment is incredibly complex. Anyone who tries to tell you that you can fix your gut with some supplement, a seven-day reset or detox is very misguided.

It's also not something that we can interpret easily, because everything is intertwined together. As humans we like to figure things out and focus on a particular species or probiotic we can use to heal some issue that's been going on.

And yes, sometimes there are pathogenic species that cause us harm, and yes, these need to be treated first. And yes, there is some good research on some probiotic species for specific medical conditions. But apart from this, we can't always focus on individual species because they in effect, all work together, so messing with one might have downstream impacts we don't yet know about or haven't considered.

They might be different strains and species of bacteria, but across all their DNA, they share functions and can in effect work together. One species produces something that another one can utilise and so on, thus really highlighting the delicate balance of the whole system.

The whole system works as a community. Much like a rainforest. If we introduce a non-native plant or insect species or build a dam, we disrupt the whole ecosystem. Because everything was in balance before. The plants and animals worked together and shared resources to make it work. With a new insult to this ecosystem, things might be considerably out of balance for some time and may never get back to a harmonious state. If we work at simplifying our diet and feeding our bacteria the types of foods, food components and fibres we know are beneficial, then we end up feeding all the beneficial species at the same time, which supports all the downstream activities that we hadn't considered but are also likely beneficial, since longer-term, epidemiological studies (not looking at the gut microbiome) support fibre intake from fruits and vegetables and whole grains, with significant health benefits and longevity. We can work towards getting our bacterial profiles back to this harmonious state.

Focusing on doing this has so many benefits you might not have even considered. Yes, your gut will work better. But when your gut is working well, your blood sugar control is improved, your cholesterol levels improve, your blood pressure improves, your sleep improves, you feel better, you can do some more activity, you are more productive and your mood is better.

See how the small changes stack up and lead to bigger ones?

In isolation, they seem almost silly. But at the end of three to four months, when you've stacked up a whole series of changes, your whole life has turned around for the better.

CHAPTER 8

Where are you at...Really?

WHAT IS THE STATE OF YOUR GARDEN?

Before you start on your inner and outer changes, it is a really good idea to hold yourself accountable, be honest and make a clear picture of where you are at. We can't change what we don't acknowledge, right?

There are a couple of ways we can do this when it comes to your health and gut health.

1. Acknowledge how you talk to yourself (chapter 1), is it kind and one of wonder in our masterpiece of our human body? If not, write those sticky notes and put them on your mirror. Remind yourself daily that you are much more than what the scales say or what social media tells us we must look like.
2. What is your gut health like currently? We can do some very simple assessments, which can help us track where we are at.

Stool form and consistency are quite well correlated with markers of gut health (9–11). How do we measure stool form and consistency then I hear you asking? Prepare to be enlightened by a poo chart.

Bristol Stool Chart

TYPE 1	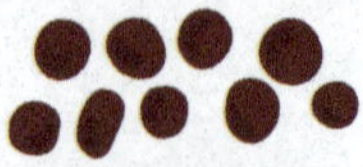	Separate hard lumps
TYPE 2	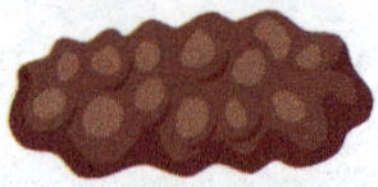	Lumpy and sausage like
TYPE 3	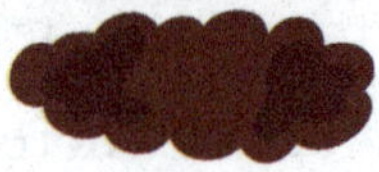	Sausage shape with cracks in the surface
TYPE 4	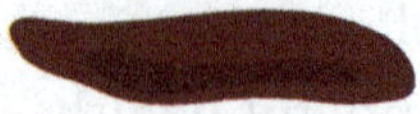	Smooth, sausage shape
TYPE 5	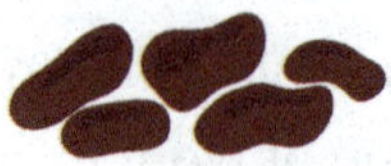	Soft blobs with clear edges
TYPE 6	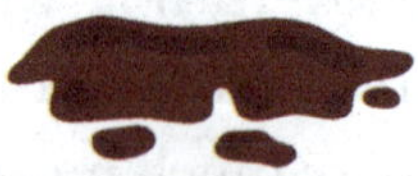	Mushy consistency, ragged edges
TYPE 7	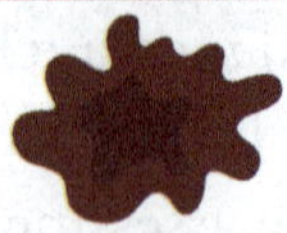	Liquid, no solid pieces

Your aim is to have a number 4-shaped bowel movement. If it is on the harder side, i.e. 1-3, then it is likely you haven't been eating enough fibre, drinking enough water, or possibly both.

If you regularly have type 6-7, then you should probably see a health professional first, because there can be some other medical conditions which cause this. It might indicate you are not absorbing things properly, but it also likely means your gut bacteria haven't had enough time to do their job properly. Once these are ruled out, we can definitely work on this to try and increase the fermentation happening, which might help slow things down.

So, how often should we be having these type 4 bowel movements? You can very easily test your current transit time at home, and in fact, it's a good one to do BEFORE you make any of the changes in this book, because it will give you a baseline value on which to base some of your improvement.

This recipe is the one used in a scientific research study, I just adapted it slightly so you only need to eat 1 muffin instead of 2 (they are quite sweet) (10).Remember to take note of the entry time… and await the exit time, to record your "transit time". The average transit in this study was around 28 hours, but values on the lower side of this were associated with better markers of gut health and an overall healthier index of gut microbiome composition. We don't want food hanging around in our colon for too long, because it gives toxins and bacteria too long to potentially cause damage to our colonic cells, but we also need the food to be in there for long enough to ferment and get broken down properly, so we can benefit from all the good things that the gut bacteria do. It's a fine balance.

If you'd rather not make actual muffins to test your transit time, you can also use something like corn kernels (corn on the cob) because these have a habit of coming out looking just like they went in (although the starch inside gets digested, they just fill up again with digestive juices). Keep in mind that because corn contributes fibre, it might actually give you a faster transit time result than you actually have. As long as you use the same test at the start and finish though, you can still get a valid result.

3. How much dietary fibre are you eating currently? This one is difficult to estimate, so I recommend tracking this one for a day or two. You will need

to find a calorie-tracking app which also reports fibre, in Australia I recommend one called Easy Diet Diary, but there are plenty of others which will do the job here. If you pop back to the chapter on dietary fibres, we talk more about this there.

4. How much ultra-processed food are you actually eating? I help you work out how to calculate this in Chapter 19, but being honest with yourself upfront about what percentage of your current diet comes from these foods will help you acknowledge where you are at, because these foods may be contributing quite significantly all by themselves to any gut issues you may be having.

5. What is your current level of gut comfort? There are plenty of questionnaires which are more validated than this basic question, but this is a really good place to start. You already know if you are feeling bloated and uncomfortable, so you certainly don't need a fifty question tool to tell you this. Give yourself a rating on your digestive comfort. If you feel a bit bloated and uncomfortable some or all of the time, then make sure you capture this and score yourself closer to 10. As you make a few dietary changes and add a bit more dietary fibre and add a few lifestyle modifications,

you might notice that this actually improves quite quickly.

You can use this table or make your own to track your baseline and your changes each week/fortnight/month as you go through this book. There are no rules for the timelines here, it is your diet, and you need to be the master of it.

	My current me	Me in _____ months time
Self-Talk How are you speaking to yourself when it comes to your body?		
Gut Health What is your current level of discomfort (1-10, 10 being high levels of discomfort)		
Bristol Stool Chart Number		
Transit Time		
Dietary fibre intake (g)		

% Ultra-processed foods		
Making 1 change at a time Remember these changes can be diet OR lifestyle-related.	Include your plan on how you will achieve this, with plans A, B and C (Chapter 7).	
1st Change		
2nd Change		
3rd Change		
4th Change		
5th Change		
6th Change		
7th Change		
8th Change		
9th Change		
10th Change		
11th Change		
12th Change		

245 g Plain Flour
15 g Baking Powder
200g white sugar
100g Canola Oil
230g Water
1 tsp Vanilla Essence
12g ROYAL BLUE food colour
(Available Kitchen Warehouse)

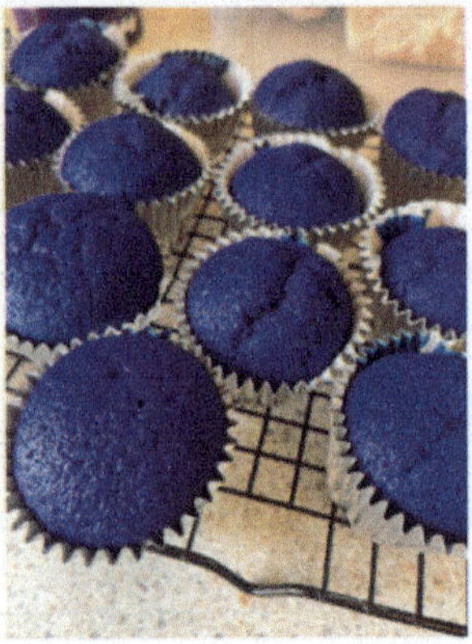

Pre heat the oven to 170 C
Combine flour, baking powder and sugar in a large bowl
In a separate bowl, combine sunflower oil, water and vanilla extract
Form a well in the centre of the dry ingredients and add the wet
Add the blue dye
Carefully measure out to exactly 12 Muffins (it's science)
Bake for 24-26 minutes, or until a skewer comes out clean.
Remember to note the time when you eat one!

CHAPTER 9

Our Brain and our Gut are Friends

THE TREES COMMUNICATE WITH EACH OTHER

The gut and the brain are two separate organ systems in our body, so it seems a bit unreal that they can "talk" to each other. When I first learned about this my eyes looked like a kid in a candy store "this is so cool!" [Science is amazing people].

There isn't some magic witchcraft happening. We now know that there are a couple of main ways that the gut and brain communicate (12):

1. Via the nervous system directly. There are nerve endings throughout our digestive system, so these are the direct and most obvious links back to the brain. The branch of the nervous system that is in this area is called the vagus nerve. If you've heard this term, it refers to the tree branch of our whole nervous system that connects to our digestive system. These nerves can control things like pain

sensitivity, the way our muscles move the food through the system and the release of other hormones and digestive juices. The vagus nerve can sense the composition of the microbiome because of the way it is embedded in the digestive tract even though it is not in direct contact with the gut microbiome itself. Most of the nerve endings in the gut are directed back to the brain (around 80% of them), but 20% of the nerve endings are for communication from the brain to the digestive tract (13). The really cool thing about these 20% of nerve fibres going this way, is that they can change microbiome composition. Not directly, but by changing the inflammatory profile via altering the ability of the junctions between cells to be stuck together. So, this really highlights the sheer power we have with just our mind.

2. Via the metabolites and hormones. Some of the molecules produced by gut bacteria, as they eat the leftover food products, enter our bloodstream. Some of these are small enough to cross the very strict barrier the brain has covering it. When these enter the brain, they help to maintain things in balance. These metabolites, and specifically short-chain fatty acids, also help to control the release of serotonin from the gut. Serotonin is one of our body's feel-good hormones, and approxi-

mately 95% of it originates from the gut (14). So, when I talk about eating well to feel good, I quite literally mean it! It's not just a mindset thing, food quite literally impacts how we feel due to the link with the bacteria, the products they produce and then in turn the feel-good hormones we produce. The short-chain fatty acids produced when the gut bacteria eat fibres, are a really crucial part of the way that the gut-brain-axis operates. Short-chain fatty acids are associated with reducing brain inflammation and degeneration, and it might also explain why we have such high prevalences of cognitive decline in the elderly. The science in this area is fascinating and demonstrates how cleverly our body has evolved (12,13,15,16) to live harmoniously with our gut friends. So, if you've noticed you don't feel good, don't feel productive, or don't feel like doing much after a few days of eating really poorly, this is in part why.

This is also why, when we start to eat better, we feel better! We feel more productive, we have more energy. Life is good. We also sleep better. Melatonin, the sleep hormone, also partly originates from the gut (17–19), so getting things in better balance in the gut can give us back some more refreshing zzz.

> The short-chain fatty acids produced from the bacterial consumption of fibre can also regulate processes like our blood sugar regulation and cholesterol, so there are many more functions than just supporting our mental well-being, but the mental aspect of what they do is very exciting.

You've probably already worked out that being stressed can influence your gut. Sometimes when we are really anxious in certain situations, we get diarrhoea. This is a direct influence of the brain communicating with the gut and changing the muscular contractions going on in there because of the anxiety. This has a flow on effect to our microbiome composition too.

The digestive tract is inside our body, but it is part of the outside world, rather than part of our body per se. The body has systems in place to protect us from this outside world, from the bits and pieces of broken-down foods, acids and bacteria that are part of this area. The mucus layer that lines the digestive tract is part of this protection system. Stress can directly influence the thickness of this mucus layer, by changing the activity of the cells that make the mucus. If the mucus layer is too thin, we can get what's called leaky gut, and this can trigger systemic low-grade inflammation. This is part of the reason why other illnesses often get worse when we are stressed (16).

The intricate communication systems between the gut and the brain can also regulate our appetite and hunger signals. Having an awareness of the role of this system can really help us make more informed decisions about how we eat.

It is well reported in the scientific literature that people gain less weight over time the more dietary fibre they consume (20), and this makes perfect sense, because fibre is really filling. Fruits, vegetables, whole grains and legumes take up a lot of space in our gut. Partly because they contain a lot of water, and partly because they are high in fibre. The fibres found in these foods can regulate our appetite by stimulating the production of short chain fatty acids, which in turn influence the production of "hunger hormones" (21). One of the signals to our brain that we are not hungry is GLP-1 (which is now sold as a weight loss drug, Ozempic or Weygovy). This hormone is naturally secreted by cells of the intestinal tract in response to various nutritional triggers, one of which is one that has also been shown to be increased naturally by increasing fibre intake (via the production of short-chain fatty acids) (21). Keep in mind there are other hormones which influence our hunger signals too, as with most things in the human body it is not a straightforward pathway. Another hormone called PYY was recently demonstrated to be specifically stimulated via the consumption of a high-fibre meal (22), showing the unique and intricate balance of fibre, other nutrients, appetite and our hunger.

If we know that changing a few things in our diet is going to improve the communication system and we know how and why it happens, then it makes it easier to get through those first few days when the change might seem hard. Keeping the end goal in mind AND only going slowly with our changes makes it much more doable.

Have a think about your current stress levels, your diet and your lifestyle generally. What are a couple of the biggest things in your life right now that are stressful? Job, children, housing stress, financial stress, etc. Some of these are hugely stressful but might pass quickly, others are prolonged stressors. Which category do yours fall into?

One of the purposes of working on our food intake and other food components is to improve the communication from our gut to our brain.

What about the communication from our brain to our gut?

This is something that supplement companies don't mention when they sell you their expensive products, but this is one of the key pieces to the puzzle of getting your gut health to a point where you are comfortable and happy.

This can also be a lot more difficult to shift than our diet! Diets and what we choose to eat can be altered quite quickly. But the way we think, the way we react and the mindset we have are a lot more difficult. You have arrived here because you wanted to do something different and take a different path with your health, so you've already taken the biggest step. The mental journey of what we do here can take a lot longer than this book. So please be kind to yourself. This is an evolving process.

There are three important points to remember.

1. Eating food is not about how we look. We eat for fuel, to feed our bacteria, to feel GOOD! How we look is the "side effect" of what happens on the inside.
2. We may not have control over some of the circumstances in our lives, but we can choose how we respond to these.
3. We are so privileged to have this choice to work on ourselves and our diet. To have so much abundance around us that we get to make this choice. Keep your perspective as one of gratefulness. I am grateful to have the resources to work on my physical and mental health.

There is some really good evidence for the use of mindfulness, breathing exercises and meditation for improving mood. There's also a link between the gut microbiome and mood. So, let's work on both at the same time. A small study from India has shown significant improvements in gastrointestinal symptoms after practising meditation for 50 days (23). This research, which is looking at the communication going back the other way from brain to gut, is still in the early days specifically for showing changes to gut microbiome composition. Another small study of elderly patients with cognitive decline, showed that performing daily mindfulness training for nine months, was associated with increased cognitive capacity and that this was associated with differences in the gut microbiome (24). Although there are lots of potential limitations with studies like these, we have to be careful that patients don't also change their diets for example, it does give us a pretty good indication that yes, the brain has the power to change the composition of the gut microbiome. This is why I love what I do, so cool!

I've never been one to be able to do meditation. I'm a high achiever, who has always found it difficult to focus and to be honest, I didn't think I needed it. And I think I'm not alone in thinking this. There are many other people that put this in the too hard or I don't need it basket.

But I'd like you to keep an open mind here, because it can quite literally change many things in your life, your gut is only one part of this. Better decisions get made in ALL areas of our lives when we are not operating from a place of stress and worry. This doesn't just apply to food.

This brings us to your homework for today.

I want to do a bit of Google searching for yourself. Do some research on breathing exercises and/or meditation. I want you to find one that you like. They are both very effective at calming the nervous system, so it is more about finding one that suits you than me telling you which one to do. I want you to find one that you can do for 5-15 minutes per day. Whether it is two x 5 minutes or one 15 minutes it doesn't matter. What is important is that you are taking some time out for yourself. You are taking some time to calm your nervous system and you are taking the time to work on your brain-to-gut connection.

Also remember that you might NOT feel like you are "good" at doing these, especially at the beginning. That is normal too! Relaxing and learning to relax without all the distractions of modern life takes time. You need to expect that it might take you a while to learn to get into the swing of it. I've been doing meditation for a while now, and I still have days here and there where I struggle to concentrate or find it difficult to relax. But it doesn't matter really, because what is important is that I recognise it wasn't quite my day, and I still feel good that I took the time out for myself regardless.

Breathing exercises are easy to fit into your day and can be done while riding on public transport. There are a few apps which help give you the counting component, so you know when you breathe in, hold, and breathe out. There are many variations of breathing exercises. For example, there is what's called the physiological "sigh", which is where you breathe in for 3, and breathe out for 6. There's box breathing, where you breathe in for 5, hold for 5, breathe out for 5 and hold for 5. These are the most common and probably the most effective, but there are also many others. The timers that go along with some of these breathing exercises are fabulous for busy minds, because your mind can wander a bit, but when that ding goes, you are brought back quickly to what you are meant to be doing.

There is also a lot of choice for mediation. If you are like me and have a busy mind, then a guided meditation where you visualise a certain scene might be a good place to start because it gives your mind something to do. If you're worried about falling asleep while you do one of these, then try sitting up when doing it or make yourself slightly uncomfortable, so it is not quite so easy to drop off. There are also plenty of meditations on Spotify or YouTube which are free, so jump on and have a look and find something you like.

After you've decided which option you want to try, your task for today is to start relaxing those gut nerves by doing some breathing or meditation. Fifteen minutes a day is what we should aim for. Headphones are great if you need to block out the noise of your house while you do it. Explain to your family what you are up to and ask them to respect your need for fifteen minutes of peace. I tell my teenagers I am on DND for 15 minutes [which is do not disturb in teenage speak, but they get it, and it works].

CHAPTER 10

Why Getting Outside is Part of the Plan

PILLAR FOUR, THE ENVIRONMENT

Okay before you stop reading and think that this doesn't matter, just keep an open mind here. Science has been giving us some pretty awesome findings lately about the benefits of being outside, for our gut AND mental health, so let's delve into that a little more.

Humans and nature have evolved together. It makes sense that our body has subconsciously developed a need and desire to be out in nature.

While there is a lot of research about environmental exposure in early life and the shaping of the gut microbiome, there is not a lot of literature about adult exposure and how this can benefit our gut directly. BUT, there is considerable evidence that nature exposure can improve six areas of our life directly, which is likely partly or mostly mediated via changes in our gut microbiome (25):

1. Our Stress Levels

Cortisol is one of our stress hormones. The evidence is very clear that exposure to nature lowers our stress hormones. Cool, hey? Now lowering of these stress hormones is also going to calm down the communication path between the brain and the gut. So, this is an amazing benefit with many flow-on effects.

2. Mood

Nature can reduce depressive mood, even following short-term exposure to the natural environment. I think we all know within ourselves we feel better if we've been out in nature, for a walk or a swim at the beach, etc. But this is really important if you're struggling with motivation. Get yourself outside for a while. Find a park. Go sit there or walk there for a bit. The water is my happy place. If I ever need a mood boost, then a dip in the ocean or a swim in the pool really hits the spot for me. On the days when I can't be bothered exercising, the pool can always turn me around. I just need to get myself out of my head and get there.

3. Cognitive Function

A growing number of studies have found that exposure to natural environments compared with urban environments is associated with improved attention, executive function and perceived restorativeness (25–30). These studies have found statistically significant associations with positive cognitive outcomes, even after short periods of time spent in natural environments.

4. Immune Function

In Japan, forest bathing (we might call this having a swim in a dam or lake in the bush) has been positively associated with human immune function (29). A study was conducted in which subjects completed a three-day/two-night bathing trip to forest areas, and blood and urine were sampled on days two and three of the trip. After the trip, it was found that the mean values of natural killer cells (which play a major role in the immune system) and natural killer cell activity were higher on forest bathing days compared with control days. This effect persisted for 30 days after the trip. A potential pathway for improved immune function is exposure to a substance emitted by plants and trees to protect themselves from harmful insects and germs, which could decrease stress hormones in the human body and increase natural killer cell activity. Additionally, the findings indicated that a day trip to a forest park also increased the levels of intracellular anti-cancer proteins.

5. Sleep

There is only preliminary evidence in this area, but increased exposure to green space during the day is associated with better sleep quality during the night. More green exposure was associated with a lower risk of short sleep duration (31). Now this might be due to a lot of things, but I want you to think about the days that you are outside for a lot of the day, how tired are you?

6. Blood Pressure

A combined study (examining 52 other studies) on the physiological effects of nature therapy and forest walking, and found overwhelming evidence that blood pressure levels decreased when participants were exposed to a natural environment (28). Decreases in both systolic and diastolic blood pressure levels were observed across young healthy populations, as well as populations with hypertension. This suggests that forest walking may lead to a state of physiological relaxation. The authors found that both systolic and diastolic blood pressure taken in the forest environment were significantly lower than in non-forest environments.

The summary here is that being out in nature, in some way shape or form is hugely beneficial. Whether or not some of these mechanisms work via the gut remains to be explored, but they WILL impact the gut indirectly, via that very effective gut-brain communication system.

If we feel better our gut feels better and then the positive reinforcement can continue. Now that we've delved into the why, we can work on the doing part. One of the things on your to-do list each day this week, should be to include at least 10 minutes outside.

It's always more successful if it's stacked onto some other activity. I always prefer to do my exercise outside. So, I tick two boxes when I do that. You could catch up with a friend for a walk and tick off three things! Being outside, being social AND doing some exercise. Smashing goals here.

CHAPTER 11

Our Bacteria Need Friends Too

PILLAR FOUR: THE ENVIRONMENT

There is a social side of the gut microbiome. Who would have thought these single-celled little critters liked having friends?

This is a completely fascinating area of science. Diet is the biggest driver of microbiome composition, but there are other areas of our life which we might not expect, which can also influence our gut.

Science has known for a long time that altering the gut microbiome can alter behaviour and there are many rodent studies showing the effects of this, as well as some pretty convincing evidence in humans from what we know of mental health disorders.

But what about the other direction? Can our social interactions play a role in the types of bacterial species that live in our colon? My science brain says well, yes, of course, it can and it likely should. When we interact socially, we often go to different environments (different bacterial loads), interact with different people, hug them, share food with them, etc. (different bacterial load) and eat foods we might not normally.

Some of the longest-living societies on earth, yes they have an amazing diet, and yes, they are much more active than us, but they also have large, connected social groups and often gather for meals together.

Rodent studies clearly show us that the social network of the mouse is strongly predictive of their gut microbiome composition, so there is no reason to think that this would also not apply to humans (32). Some of the oldest citizens of the Guangxi province in China are the ones with more "youthful" microbiomes (33), suggesting that sharing gut microbiomes in social situations may indeed impact our health and longevity.

A smaller study looking at family dynamics and gut microbiomes showed that "human interactions, especially sustained, close marital relationships, influence the gut microbiota (34)".

Research also tells us that people with larger social networks have more diverse gut microbiomes (35).

While environmental factors like social networks are important for contributing to our gut microbiome composition, I don't even need to spell this out, but social connectedness is also really important for our well-being generally. Having connected networks is a very strong predictor of mental health (36), so we win in many areas of health when we have stronger social networks.

The take-home message from this is that being with family and friends is good for us for more reasons than we might think.

As a parent, I completely understand how difficult it is fitting all these things into our schedule, but we can certainly get clever about doing it so that we get the best of all of it. We'll talk about exercise in the next chapter, but exercise is a great way to combine a few of these lifestyle factors together, because it is easy when we do things with friends, and/or we do them outside.

Shift your mindset about catching up with your friends and move to doing something healthy together, like a walk on the beach or a game of golf or something outside. You get the benefit of the activity and the social catch-up all in one.

CHAPTER 12

The Journey to Poop

WATERING YOUR GARDEN

The term gut microbiome or gut microbiota describes the collection of bugs (bacteria, archaea, viruses and yes, some fungi) that live in our colon. How and why are they there though?

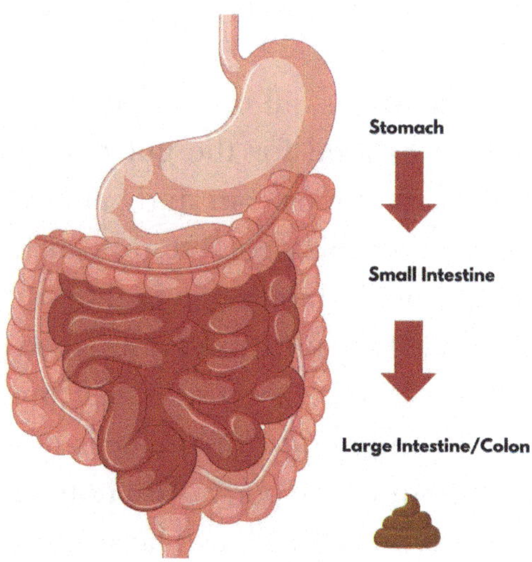

When we eat, the small intestine is where our human cells take up whatever they can, in terms of energy and nutrients. These little molecules of food (which are all broken down by now into very, very small particles) pass into the bloodstream and are delivered to the rest of the body. We will go into this in a bit more detail shortly. The cells lining our small intestine specialise in taking up all the bits and pieces at different rates and passing it through to the bloodstream only when the work is complete enough that it passes the test of the little transporters that allow it through to the other side. Very clever really and beautifully engineered to ensure our survival.

The one thing to remember is that the process, like most production lines, is not 100% efficient. Some things that maybe should have been absorbed were not, because of the fact that they were stuck in the matrix of the food, or they passed through too quickly, or the little transporters couldn't take it all up.

All of these leftovers, all of the food our human cells can't use, end up as food for the gut microbiome in the colon. It's like our compost bin and rainforest all at the same time. A very complex ecosystem, which has evolved to live in harmony with the human body.

The bacteria eat the fibres and other food components that are "leftovers", and in return, they produce many, many beneficial compounds for the cells of our digestive tract, but also for our entire body. Also note that many detrimental products can be produced here too, and these can increase dramatically if our gut runs short on the preferred food source, which is primarily fibres.

Some of these beneficial compounds are called short-chain fatty acids. Remember this, we will be talking about these again in more detail later. They are some of the key superpowers of the gut microbiome!

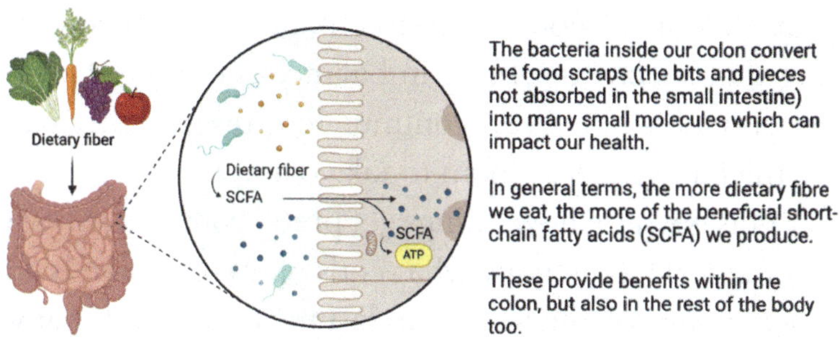

Figure 1. Created in BioRender. Genoni, A. (2025) https://BioRender.com/1bw370k.

So, if our bacterial friends eat fibre as their preferred dish of choice, then what is fibre exactly?

When you hear the term dietary fibre (or see it on a food label), you might think it is one type of chemical compound. It is one word, but a large group of compounds with hundreds of different combinations.

The two things they have in common are 1; they are not taken up by human cells in the small intestine 2; they ONLY come from the cell wall of the plants. You have to eat the cells and the cell walls to get it!

Here is the cool thing about fibre. Each type of fibre is the favourite dish for a particular species of beneficial bacteria. Much like your cat, if you have one at home. They are a bit precious, have their favourite food and they'll only eat something different if they are majorly starving.

The colonic bacteria, however, are made up of not just beneficial bacteria. The rainforest in the gut is made up of all sorts of good (and potentially bad) species. The thing that keeps everything in balance is feeding the good guys enough so they can continue to grow and thrive and give the bad guys less room to take over.

This is where now, things get pretty complex. After we eat a meal, what actually what ends up in the colon is a little percentage of whatever that last meal was, and that will be a complex mixture of fibres, undigested carbohydrates, proteins, fats (and the bile acids that are used for the digestive process) was comprised of. So, what if that meal was a lot of fat and/or protein? The types of bacteria that thrive on this as a food source are not necessarily the type of bacteria we would term "good guys". These ones take the fat (which is bound up with bile) and metabolise the bile into secondary bile acids (some of which are toxic), and the protein, into phenols, cresols, ammonia and other compounds not desirable in the colonic environment (37). In addition, protein-loving bacterial species can thrive here, especially when we talk about consuming large amounts of animal protein (38). This is why I'm firstly more concerned about you eating enough fibre to balance any of this out, and secondly, not overdoing the protein. Especially, the animal protein. Plant proteins happen to be quite well bound up with beneficial fibres and polyphenols and don't appear to have the same impact on altering populations of beneficial gut bacteria (39).

Having some different types of fibres with all of our meals means we specifically stimulate the beneficial bacterial species and provide less chance for some of the less beneficial ones to grow. Science tells us that having a lot of different types of bacteria in our gut is a good thing, so then it now seems obvious that we need to eat a wide variety of fibres to feed a wide variety of the good guys in our gut.

The recommendations are to eat about 25-30g of fibre per day, but this is actually very low compared to other hunter-gatherer societies who can easily eat upwards of 50g (40). Our gut bacteria and digestive systems have evolved to eat much more fibre than we currently eat. We know that the more fibre we eat, the less weight gain we have as we get older, the less likely we are to get cardiovascular disease, diabetes and many types of cancers. This is purely due to giving our bacteria more food to eat so they can in return support our health with many beneficial compounds.

One of my aims for my clients when I work with them, is to get them eating the recommended intake of fibre as an absolute minimum. But we don't want to do this all at once, because this is not comfortable or sustainable. [Change too many things at once in your diet at your own peril (or that of your toilet)].

This is where my one-change-at-a-time philosophy really comes into its own.

I don't normally recommend tracking your calorie intake, but I do want you to get a feel for where you are at with your fibre intake. Your task for the next few days is to pick one 24-hour period, and record everything you eat and drink for the day. You'll need to use an app like Easy Diet Diary (this is an Australian based-app, but there are other good ones out there) because this one gives you fibre information in the free version.

I want you to hold yourself accountable to yourself. How much fibre are you actually eating in your diet right now? Make a note of it somewhere, and we can revisit this again in a few weeks, to see if you've been able to increase it. After you've got your list of foods eaten in the day, take a look at the big picture. What sorts of foods are providing the fibre? Now that we just learned we need a variety of fibre, examine your intake. Is all your fibre coming from one place?

If you just found that all your fibre came from wholegrain breads or cereals, then let's look at adding in some fruit or vegetable/s over the coming weeks to give your gut the diversity it needs. But read the next chapter first before you try and overwhelm yourself with too many changes.

CHAPTER 13

The Nitty-Gritties of Digestion

WATERING THE GARDEN A BIT MORE

In the last chapter, we had a very brief overview of the digestive process to give us an idea of how things end up in the colon for bacterial dinner.

It's also useful to have a more in-depth understanding of how your human cells make use of the food we eat. Understanding how your body works better is part of the empowerment and confidence-building process.

Approach this chapter with a bit of wow, not a bit of boring. Your perspective on this matters because approaching it with a bit of "OMG this is boring" is going to leave you in the same place you were before you even picked up this book.

When we have an appreciation for how specialised all of our cells are and we can step back and have some wonder about what an absolute masterpiece of engineering our body is, this is when we can truly love and appreciate ourselves.

Loving our body and what it does behind the scenes gives us more of a reason to nurture it.

DIGESTION STARTS IN THE MOUTH

For our body to take up molecules of food and turn them into new cells or energy, all of those food particles need to be broken down at the cellular level.

This process is both mechanical via chewing and muscular contractions of the digestive tract, and chemical, via the secretion of digestive juices.

In the mouth, we obviously chew our food, which starts the process of breaking things apart. Our saliva wets the food and our saliva contains amylase, which is an enzyme to commence the breakdown of starches.

THINGS RAMP UP IN THE STOMACH

I think we all know that the contents of the stomach are pretty acidic. The acid load here serves a couple of purposes. First, acid is good at dissolving things. It has this effect in the stomach too. It is a very good way to break down food into smaller particles. The second purpose is to regulate the bacterial load entering the rest of the digestive tract (41). The acid here doesn't kill everything, but it certainly does a good job of reducing the overall load that makes it through the system. Which is a good thing, otherwise we might find ourselves quite sick more often. The stomach is also very muscular. The contractions are in all directions, to really mix the food around and ensure that it is well mixed with the acid before proceeding on its journey.

Food particles are not absorbed into the body from the stomach (except alcohol), the purpose of the stomach is to mix it up, commence the breakdown process and get it ready for further digestion in the small intestine. Alcohol is the only exception here, because the alcohol molecule is so small and it is lipid soluble, it can bypass our usual checks and balances and diffuses all by itself across the stomach wall and into the blood supply. Hence, we can notice quickly the effects of alcohol.

Food usually spends around twenty minutes in the stomach, before being drip-fed to the small intestine.

The stomach is well designed for the acid load, with specialised cells and a thick layer of mucus to protect the cells, but the rest of the digestive tract can be a bit vulnerable to this high acid load. So, there are a few checkpoints (sphincters) which regulate how much and when food is allowed to proceed past to the next stop on the journey.

THE SMALL INTESTINE: WHERE THE MAGIC HAPPENS

The acidic chyme as it is now called, is slowly passed into the small intestine. The pancreas and liver (via the gall bladder) are now in charge of helping out here, secreting a whole host of other digestive enzymes into the small intestine. These enzymes and bile acids happen to be quite basic, so they start to neutralise the acid, which makes sure our small intestine does not get toasted from all the acid.

FATS

Bile is an important part of fat digestion. Bile is like a soap. It coats the fat molecules, so they don't re-conglomerate back together. Bile is a greenish compound and part of the reason our poop is brown (aren't you glad you now know this?).

Bile is responsible for ensuring the fat stays in small enough particles, then other enzymes from the pancreas (lipases) break the fat into its components. Fats are technically triglycerides (see picture below), which means they are molecules containing three fatty acid tails and a glycerol backbone. These need to be disassembled before our cells can take them all up. Just like taking apart IKEA furniture. Because of the three fatty acid tails (which can be quite long), the amount of energy these can provide the body is quite large. This is why fats are more calorie dense than carbohydrates or proteins.

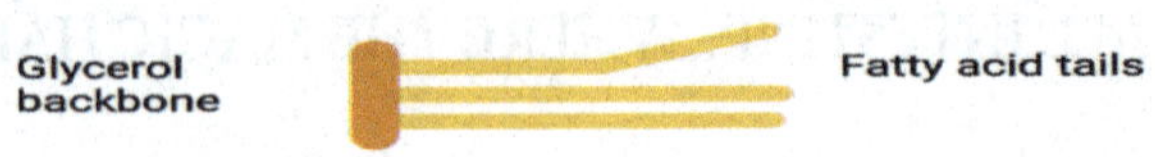

Figure 2. Created in BioRender. Genoni, A. (2025) https://BioRender.com/6k38chw

The cool thing about fat digestion (specifically, the triglycerides), is that the fats don't go directly to our bloodstream. They are especially transported via the lymphatic system first, then to the bloodstream. The body has very strict rules for transporting fats around the body too, which are part of what is measured when you have your cholesterol levels sampled.

One of the things tested in a standard cholesterol panel, is triglycerides. Now you know where these come from. The amount of these that stay in your bloodstream is important, because if we aren't clearing them out effectively, it can interrupt many other processes and place us at increased risk of metabolic and cardiovascular dysfunction.

If you are exercising and eating well, your muscles and liver will use these triglycerides for energy. Otherwise, they are very efficiently stored as fat (sorry).

Fat digestion doesn't end when the triglycerides are taken up. Because there were a lot of bile acids used to help with the process and because this product takes a lot of manufacturing time, the body tries to recycle this. Some of these bile acids are also reabsorbed in the small intestine after fat the were accompanying is gone, but some bile passes through to the colon.

One of the components of bile is cholesterol, so if you've seen or heard that oat fibre can reduce cholesterol levels, this is how it works. The beta-glucans in oats, bind up the bile and force it through to the colon, where it is excreted. Because it reduces our total pool of cholesterol in the body, our blood cholesterol levels drop. There's actually a lot of research around bile acids at the moment, because it seems they are not just innocuous helpers to the digestive process, but they are in fact signalling molecules for many processes both within and outside the digestive tract (42).

If we end up with an excess of bile in the colon (not bound to a fibre), some of these are consumed by bacterial species and turned into more toxic compounds, called secondary bile acids. Not really desirable, because these are linked with colon cancer formation (43). This is also why I'm not really an advocate for high-fat diets. Firstly, the fat displaces other nutrients like fibre from your diet, but secondly, you'll end up with high amounts of secondary bile acids (and many other compounds related to the increased protein intake) in the colon.

PROTEINS

Protein digestion is also like disassembling IKEA furniture. Proteins are chains of amino acids joined together. The configuration of the amino acid sequences are different, depending on the protein source. Some will have more of specific amino acids than others.

When I did my undergraduate degree, it was thought that plant proteins didn't provide all of the essential amino acids; however, we now know this is incorrect. Plants might be deficient in certain amino acids, but different plants have different ones missing, so as long as you eat a variety of plants, you will still get all of the required amino acids.

So, the role of the body is to disassemble all the protein we eat into amino acids. The amino acids can then be used to reassemble different proteins in the body. All of our enzymes, blood haemoglobin, muscle cells, skin proteins, etc., are made of amino acids, and these are replaced on a very regular basis.

The stomach acid begins the dismantling process, but it is the proteases secreted by the pancreas which are like the Allen key to making sure the proteins are down to small individual amino acids or small chains called peptides.

The most important thing I want to point out here is that eating protein in excess of your requirements does not mean this extra protein magically ends up on your muscles. If you're not stressing your muscles and telling them to grow (i.e. by using them), then you guessed it, that excess protein is burned as energy or stored as fat (sorry).

CARBOHYDRATE DIGESTION

While we are on the theme of disassembling IKEA furniture, carbohydrates are exactly the same. Carbohydrates are often called sugars, and the reason for this is that they are actually chains of sugars joined together.

There are three simple single sugar molecules: glucose, fructose and galactose.

Table sugar is a disaccharide (meaning two sugars), comprising glucose + fructose.

Lactose (milk sugar) is also a disaccharide, glucose + galactose.

Starch is a very long chain of glucose molecules and can be 1,000 or more glucose units joined together.

Our human digestive enzymes are specialised at breaking apart these bonds between the sugars. We need a special enzyme to break the bond between the milk sugars (lactase), and some people genetically don't produce much or any of this.

If this is you, you've likely worked this out by the unavoidable stomach cramps that happen after eating milk or ice cream ☺. Cheese and yoghurts are often better tolerated in these cases, because the fermentation of these products reduces the lactose present to start with.

Why do we get the stomach cramps then if it's just a simple sugar we are not digesting?

These simple sugars are meant to be mostly all absorbed in the small intestine. If they happen to make it through to the colon, they first attract a lot of water and secondly, the bacteria in the colon think there's a party happening. So, you'll likely get rapid fermentation at the start of the colon, which can cause a lot of pain and gas, plus diarrhoea from the additional water that ended up there. Not a great or comfortable combo.

The simple sugars or the broken-down carbohydrates into simple sugars are taken up in the small intestine by a very specialised transport system, which selectively grabs the glucose molecules from inside the small intestine and puts them into the bloodstream. Much like passing go on the Monopoly board, everything must pass through the liver first, because the blood supply heading away from the intestines makes a stop here. The liver checks things over, and detoxifies things that it needs to from our blood, before permitting it to go on its way to the rest of the body.

Glucose is the key driver of a cascade of hormonal changes that occur after we eat. Glucose in the blood triggers the pancreas to produce insulin and send it to the bloodstream. Insulin is like the "pack it away" hormone. Its goal is to clear the glucose from the blood, by sending it to the muscles, or directing it to fat storage. Getting a spike in blood glucose after you eat is completely normal! There's a lot of misinformation out there about this process. Your body was designed to eat, to get a spike in glucose and for it to fall again. There is only an issue when this process is prolonged, that is, blood sugar stays high for too long, or if insulin is not working as it should (insulin resistance). In either case, diet modification and exercise encourage the process to work a little more efficiently again. The more glucose your muscles use, the more efficient you get at putting the glucose away after you eat.

There is a limit, however, to the amount of sugar that our small intestine can take up in one go. So, if you eat a whole bag of lollies in one sitting you might exceed the capacity of the little transporters in your small intestine to absorb all the glucose and fructose. This means we will have more glucose and/or fructose ending up in the colon. Complex carbohydrates, like fibre, are preferred bacterial food, because first it is the beneficial bacteria that possess the enzymes to break these apart, and second, they take considerable time to break down, and in doing so, produce large amounts of beneficial short-chain fatty acids. The issue with simple sugars in the colon is that because they are so simple, many different bacterial species can utilise these, even the not-so-good-bacteria (44,45) and we then inadvertently feed the types of species we really don't want to be promoting in the first place.

The take-home message from this chapter, is that your body is absolutely clever and fantastic on a cellular level for all the work it does behind the scenes. Quietly chugging away, putting away all our food particles and keeping the system organised. It's mind-blowingly beautiful if you look at it in the right way.

But it's also amazingly complex. There is much science still has to learn about digestion, we are only just beginning to understand how the bile acids operate for example, and how they can also possibly regulate so many other processes in the body (42).

Wellness influencers can easily fool you with their confidence about "what they know".

Keep in mind that experts are never so confident with what they know, for a reason. We understand the deep limitations of our knowledge and we are also very quick to acknowledge what we don't know.

This is really something to use to spot an actual expert from a fake one. Especially when they are so confidently telling you something about digestion, or blood sugar control, or insulin, that even "experts don't know".

CHAPTER 14

The Wonderful World of Fibre

PILLAR ONE: BACTERIAL FUEL

Now that we know that fibre specifically feeds the good guys in our colon, let's look a bit more closely at the types of fibre that contribute to good gut health. While we go through this, you might think to yourself, wow, that one gives me terrible bloating.

Fibre is actually a very similar chemical structure to carbohydrates. It's just that the joins between the sugars are a type that our human cells can't break apart. But bacteria can. Fibres are also many different lengths (like a necklace), some also are not just straight chains, but have complex branches. This changes the rate at which bacteria can eat them. Some of these compounds are soluble in water, some are not. This also changes the rate at which bacteria can eat it.

If you've heard the term FODMAP, then this stands for **F**ermentable **O**ligosaccharides, **D**isaccharides, **M**onosaccharides **A**nd **P**olyols. These are quite short-chain fibres, so they are fermented (or eaten) by bacteria very quickly. This is why they can cause symptoms if you suffer from IBS. The symptoms are also the result of the nerves in the colon being irritated, and so they can react to things that might not bother other people.

There are three main groups of compounds that fall under the definition of dietary fibre.

1. The plant cell walls. These have a really complex name called non-starch polysaccharides. This basically means that they are like starch, but not starch because the joins are different, so our human cells can't use them.

    a) These are basically the fibres from fruits and vegetables and the cell walls (husks) from whole grains.

2. Resistant oligosaccharides. Oligosaccharides are small sugars, with a join that our human cells can't use. These are found in things like garlic, onions, artichokes, beans and some dairy products. Because they are small, they are often used up quite high in the colon and may be triggering for some people.
3. Resistant starches. Starch in general CAN be utilised by our human cells. But if the chains of starch are really long, then it takes too long to access (because our human cells can only chop

> off and utilise one sugar unit at a time), and much of it is still intact when it enters the colon. Becoming bacterial lunch. This stuff is like bacteria superfood! They produce high amounts of those short-chain fatty acids when they consume this. Resistant starch is found in whole grains, root vegetables and greenish bananas.

Having a healthy gut microbiome relies on having all of these types of fibres, because remember, a diverse microbiome is a healthy one. We want to feed all of the good guys.

Because all the types of fibre are different and the location and rate at which they are fermented in the colon are different, some types (or subtypes) of fibre can irritate some people. This usually happens in conditions like IBS, where the gut has become sensitive to rapid fermentation and so the nerve endings respond accordingly, by letting you know there is pain going on in there. This usually occurs when the fermentation is rapid and in the very first part of the colon (called the proximal colon). If you decided to pick up this book because you're already struggling with IBS, then you're probably already familiar with the term "FODMAPs" and have worked out which ones don't agree with your gut.

One of the key strategies for managing symptoms is to cut down these irritating fibres. Unfortunately, science tells us that cutting these down, yes, does reduce symptoms, but it can also reduce the abundance of some of the beneficial bacteria in our colon (46). This is because they are short-chain carbohydrates, they are the preferred food source for some of the good guys that we really do like to have in our colon.

Going on a low FODMAP diet, therefore, is meant to be a short-term solution to managing symptoms. What we can do is try and reduce the sensitivity of the gut at the time of reducing the FODMAPs by increasing other, beneficial fibres. As in, increase all of our background fibre intake. Then we try re-introduction of VERY SMALL amounts of the offending FODMAPs, perhaps in combination with other, less rapidly fermentable fibre to reduce the likelihood of symptoms recurring.

I've talked to many people who've been on very long-term low FODMAP diets, and if this is you, it is great you are here so we can make sure your current gut can support your health in the long-term.

A low FODMAP diet is super useful, but only for short periods, and if you need support to re-introduce things, make sure you get it, because what we don't want is for you to end up with a less diverse microbiome over time as this might lead to other chronic health conditions.

My goal for my programme (and this book) is for you to be able to diversify your fibre intake so you can improve the diversity of your gut bacteria. In return, many of your other health markers will also improve.

The key piece of advice if you're struggling with FODMAPs that, yes, to reduce them to get your symptoms under control to start with. We then need to increase your background fibre intake from other fibres to build up the strength of your gut microbiome again. We are aiming to increase consumption of more slowly fermentable fibres and keep things moving in a comfortable way.

We then slowly introduce some of our offending triggers. But we don't do them by eating them by themselves. It can often be helpful to consume them with or directly after some higher-fibre, more slowly fermentable fibres. This way, the FODMAP is forced further down the colon to be fermented, rather than cause trouble high up in the first part of the colon.

This approach can be highly variable and very individual, so while I do recommend knowing your body and being in charge, if you are suffering from this type of problem, that you do get some professional guidance too, because it can really be a game changer for getting your food confidence back again. Plus, those beneficial bacteria that eat those FODMAPs also do good things for the rest of the body, so hopefully once we can get a small amount of these back into your diet again, you will actually notice the difference.

CHAPTER 15

Hello Farts

THE SIDE EFFECTS OF PILLAR ONE

Today we are going to delve a little deeper into getting more fibre into our diet – but doing it in a way that our gut is happy with.

A short digression first. I made a mistake when I was doing my PhD. I was asked if I could help out with science week at the primary school my kids were at. As I have three boys, what better thing to speak about than the gut and poop and farting? Primary school-aged kids love this stuff. I took my white coat and the anatomy model from the University (which we nicknamed Bob, not relevant, but you might need to know we cared about his name) and did a talk for a couple of the classes about the gut and all the wonderful bacteria that live there. We also talked about how to tell if your gut was working well after what you ate, and I happened to mention that farting meant that your good bugs were having a wonderful time and it was a good thing. This was all fun until the next day when more than a couple of parents were most unpleased with me telling their kids that farting was ok... But it really is, and I tell this story because, particularly in Australia, it is a bit taboo to talk about, and really, it should not be. We should perhaps (and maybe I should have specified to the kids) that they could probably pick the time and the place to release the gas though :0

Where does the gas come from? If you think back to your high school chemistry, as part of some chemical reactions, a gas is the by product. For example, if we add acid to a carbonate, then we get a salt and carbon dioxide. It is a similar situation in the gut. As a by-product of bacteria consuming some food sources, that various gases are produced. Such as, hydrogen, methane and hydrogen sulphide (47). The gas produced depends on the type of bacteria you have in your gut and the foods you are eating.

If you increase your fibre intake – you will get some extra gas and/or bloating for a day or two. This is normal and it is your bacteria adjusting themselves. As long as we don't increase it too rapidly – your tummy should cope just fine.

This is also why I have a very strong philosophy for one change at a time - promoting a high-fibre diet doesn't sound very appealing if you have to do it all at once and spend the week on the toilet feeling uncomfortable.

You might be asking yourself now, but where does the gas go then if we increase our fibre intake more slowly? Good question! Our gut is like a rainforest. It is a complex ecosystem of species that work together. Increasing your fibre slowly gives the ecosystem time for procedures to be put in place, so to speak, for the extra gas. This might be in the form of other species metabolising the gases or it might be that other species that don't produce gas but also feed on that fibre can have time to catch up to the party. It's all a delicate balance, and while things can adjust rapidly, often slow and steady is better.

We want to have a mix of fibres in our diet. Some from grains (and different grains), some from fruits and some from vegetables (including legumes and nuts) if you can tolerate these too.

Legumes have a bad reputation for causing gas and yes they do, but this usually happens when you aren't used to eating them and then you eat a whole can of baked beans. They are really beneficial for our gut because they contain high amounts of resistant starch, but also some of the shorter chain fibres (the FODMAPs), so they are a favourite dish for some of the most beneficial species in our gut. Legumes are also really cheap and a very good source of protein, especially the ones that are already cooked and canned. A quick rinse and they are ready to use. If you don't normally eat legumes and want to give them a try, please start with only a tablespoon or two! Some of the milder-tasting beans are things like cannellini or butter beans. Black beans are great in Mexican-style dishes, and chickpeas are fantastic in curries but can be a bit starchy and nutty.

What about really stinky gas?

I actually get asked this question a lot! This can be caused by a number of things. Foul smelling gas is most commonly caused by protein degradation (particularly animal proteins and sometimes legumes, which are high in sulphur containing amino acids) in the colon. This can happen if you had a giant steak at dinner last night, and the human cells in your small intestine might not have been able to get at all (or most of) the protein in time, and some of it ended up in the colon.

In true science style, this has actually been researched ☺. Sixteen people volunteered their flatus for a study which found that the sulphur-containing gases were the biggest contributor to smell (47). Can we just stop and give thanks to the people who donated their time (and flatus) for the good of science before we continue? The sulphur-containing gases most likely originate from overconsumption of protein, which has high amounts of sulphur-containing amino acids and/or having high abundances of bacteria that produce hydrogen sulphide gas.

If you're not familiar with this smell, then think rotten eggs. Eating more plant-fibres and resistant starches should put this back in balance, producing more hydrogen instead which does not smell nearly as bad.

I can almost hear you asking right about now...What about a fibre supplement, won't that just do the trick to fix my gut/flatus problems? We will talk some more about that in the next chapter.

CHAPTER 16

Do We Need Fibre Supplements?

WATERING THE KNOWLEDGE OF PILLAR ONE

If you follow me on social media, you will have already noticed I am not big on supplements. They are super expensive, most of us don't really know what we are getting and for many of them, science has absolutely no idea of the long-term effects.

My take-home message is always, "try food first".

However, there is a time and a place for a fibre supplement, especially if you have had ongoing gut issues or irritation. Getting things moving at the correct pace again can actually just help to restore your gut microbiome by itself.

There are three categories of supplements in the fibre category (48,49):

1. Laxatives. These irritate the digestive tract enough to stimulate the muscular contractions of the small and large intestine and do the job of "getting things moving". These are definitely only a short-term solution, and any type of long-

term use may lead to dependence on them for any type of bowel movement at all.

2. Bulking supplements (Metamucil, etc.). These are mostly insoluble fibres that are not fermented well by bacteria, but because they attract water, they do a pretty good job of getting the system going again. If you are needing to take this type of supplement regularly, then having your diet checked over is a good idea, because there is likely an easy fix or two that will mean this type of supplement is not needed.
3. Fermentable fibre supplements (slowly and rapidly fermentable fibres). These can be anything from pectin, to resistant starch, inulin, galacto-oligosaccharides or fructo-oligosaccharides.

If you've tried any of these and had success with any of them, then it is a good clue for what we need to work on in your diet. If Metamucil works for you, then it's a good sign we probably need to include more of the insoluble plant fibres in your diet.

Why can't I just take the supplement long-term?

Well, you can if you like…but here's the thing. Science has only really done shorter-term studies on many of them. So, we don't have a full understanding of modifying the gut microbiome with this sort of thing for a long–term period. Secondly, when we eat the fibre from the actual food, it is also packed up with all the other beneficial things found in that particular food. Like all the polyphenols (the colourful compounds) found in fruits, vegetables, legumes and whole grains. Plus, the type of fibre you get from actual food is balanced out with a range of fibres, so it's already like a broad-spectrum supplement by itself. It also didn't cost $80 and was only available on a 12-month subscription.

Food is way easier in the long run.

Some science does indicate that fibre supplements might be useful to help with weight loss, however. In a review of supplementation studies, it was shown that soluble fibre supplements might be useful in this area (50). However, it is very difficult to summarise fibre supplementation studies when they all use different fibre types and dosages (remember there are an awful lot of soluble fibre compounds), over different periods of time. The authors of this review also classified long-term as a period of greater than three months, so taking some type of supplement for a true long-term period, of longer than 1-2 years, might have very different impacts.

If the majority of your dietary fibre comes from food sources and you add another 3-5g from a supplement, that probably won't have too much of an impact long-term on the gut, but again, we can't really say that for sure.

I am pretty big on not wasting money on supplements. Fibre supplements, however, can have a time and a place – especially if you've had some gut issues or irritation. It can help settle things down, but ideally, we want to get back to having all of our fibre from food sources.

For patients struggling with IBS-type symptoms, things like partially hydrolysed guar gum (Sunfibre) can sometimes be useful. This type of fibre is a non-starch polysaccharide. It is very slowly fermented and can help shift the location of fermentation, of other fibres, further down the colon and make things more comfortable. We also want to support the growth of beneficial bacterial species, to reduce inflammation going forward, so including some resistant starch and whatever other fibres you can tolerate at the same time can also help to calm things down.

Resistant starch can be found in supplement form as Hi-Maize or green banana flour, and both are very high in resistant starch. This is easily added into smoothies. Just note, it can be constipating if you don't also include other sources of fibre.

If you are taking any sort of fibre supplement or just increasing your intake in general, remember you also need to increase your fluid intake. Fibre attracts water. Without enough water in your colon, your bacteria can't do their job properly, and you will get constipated.

But before you spend money on supplements it is always better to try and work on things with ACTUAL food. Whilst scientific research shows some of these supplements are fine and perhaps beneficial in the short-term, it is a reminder that we still don't have a full understanding of what we are messing with in the long-term when it comes to our gut microbiome. It's a complex ecosystem in there, and there might be downstream long-term effects we haven't discovered yet. This is why sticking to actual foods is safer in the long run.

CHAPTER 17

Bacteria Like Colours Too

PILLAR TWO: BACTERIAL "VITAMINS"

This chapter delves some more into the little details of the colourful side of food. These act sometimes like a fibre and provide food to the little guys in our gut, and sometimes they act as population modifiers, being able to regulate things without directly being bacterial food.

The most important part of this chapter is to not get caught up on the little details. This is stressful. This wastes your precious time and energy when you really should be out doing fun things or focusing some time on yourself.

It is the big picture that matters.

Yes, we need to feed our microbiome properly. Yes, eating high amounts of fibre and colourful compounds and having low amounts of ultra-processed foods and animal proteins is good too.

But should we be extreme and hung up on doing that 100% of the time? Absolutely not.

Go out for dinner with your friends. Order what you feel like. Keep the perspective. Enjoy what you are there for. The shared joy of having a meal with people you care about. One meal in the context of two- or three-week's worth of meals is not going to make much difference.

Remember, being stressed changes the gut too. Getting better gut health means putting in the work for the other areas that can also support our gut. Making some space in our heads and letting go of the stress we might be feeling about all these little things, opens us up for so much good to come in.

So, what are polyphenols? It is a complex sounding word, but in simple terms, it refers to a really big group of chemical compounds (there are hundreds of different types) produced by plants. Simplistically, plants produce these to protect themselves from all sorts of environmental stresses (51) (UV light, fungal attack, etc.).

Some of these compounds are very colourful, like in berries or cocoa, others like those found in oats are a little less intense. They are quite complex compounds with many, many different varieties.

In the plant, these compounds provide anti-oxidant, anti-bacterial, or anti-inflammatory effects, which is very cool, and so it makes sense that this might also apply to the effect on us when we eat it.

Science initially thought that these compounds provided another food source for bacteria, just like a dietary fibre, but we now understand that while some of them can be used as food and have a prebiotic effect, most influence our gut rainforest via the effects they were meant to have in the plant.

For example, the polyphenols with antioxidant properties influence the populations of bacteria in our gut because they reduce oxidative stress in the gut environment (51,52). The polyphenols with an anti-bacterial effect can directly down-regulate some of the less desirable species of bacteria in the gut. It is really interesting that the types of bacteria that these influence, are the ones that we don't really want there anyway, showing the beautiful and intricate balance that evolution has provided us with.

These compounds might be brightly coloured, but the actual amount of them in food is only small. In total, we might eat only a gram or less of these each day.

In science, to understand how things work, we need to isolate them and study them separately. This work has partly been done for many of the polyphenol compounds. But what science hasn't worked out completely, is how these polyphenol compounds benefit us when we eat them as part of a total dietary pattern. We know that populations who eat higher amounts of foods that contain them, like berries or tea, have health benefits. However, because there are a huge range of polyphenol compounds present in food/s, the mechanisms by which these benefit us are still not well understood.

If you've seen some social media on one of these polyphenol compounds and want to try taking one of them, you do need to do a bit of research. Many companies selling these types of supplements clearly spend a lot of money on marketing and advertising and as a result the product is very expensive, well-branded and in an aesthetically pleasing pack. Going on face value it is almost impossible to determine the actual quality of the product. You need to invest a little of your own time in evaluating a few things.

If you do choose to take a supplement of one of these compounds it is really important to check the dose that has been used in the clinical study, who was the target population and remember that taking these in isolation *is exactly the same as taking any other kind of drug*. There might be side effects, there might be longer-term effects we don't know about yet or an interaction with another prescribed medication you are taking. Science doesn't yet have all the answers for the huge number of these things that have made their way to the market based on short-term research in small populations.

What foods do polyphenols come in and how can we make sure we get a good range of them in our diet? If you've heard the advice before to eat the rainbow, this is perfect. Eating a rainbow really does ensure that we are consuming a broad range of polyphenols.

Different polyphenols can have specific and beneficial health effects. For example, the flavonoids found in tea and apples can help prevent cardiovascular disease and improve blood flow in our vessels (53,54), the polyphenols in vegetables are associated with reductions in cardiovascular risk in older women (55), and the polyphenols in cereals and legumes work together with the fibres in these foods to create their beneficial effect (56).

There is one type of polyphenol group that I want to specifically mention, because the traditional way of consuming this one is not in the whole food form and it still has many health benefits associated with it. I am referring to Extra Virgin Olive Oil (EVOO). It is called Extra virgin because it has not undergone any further processing other than squeezing the olives to get the oil out and then some filtering to remove the sediment. There are quite a few different polyphenols found in olives and together they are called Olive Oil Phenolic Compounds (57). Extra virgin olive oil has been part of a traditional Mediterranean diet for many generations and is part of the reason this particular dietary pattern is associated with such good health outcomes. It has been shown to reduce LDL cholesterol, reduce inflammation and increase microbial diversity in the colon (57). EVOO phenolics are unique because they have this effect without being consumed in conjunction with the fibre found in the whole food, i.e. the olives. So, olive oil is the only oil I recommend for use in cooking, salads and for dipping fresh bread into. Just remember that oils are still 100% fat, so they are still very calorie dense. A small amount used in cooking and on salads is perfect.

In summary, there is a lot of good research supporting the beneficial effect of berries, cruciferous vegetables, apples, orange vegetables and so on (58). Rather than focusing in on any one type of these, the message needs to be about variety and increasing your rainbow of consumption.

This area of research is fascinating, especially when we look at different types of polyphenols and the cool ways that they can impact our body. To make sure we get all these cool effects, we do really need to eat the rainbow. But we don't need to get caught up on amounts and different colours. Just try something new this week, add a different colour or two, to what you normally have.

If you write down everything you eat over the course of the day today, or even write it down for a couple of days, have an objective talk with yourself about your variety. If you group your fruits and vegetables by colours, then how many colours did you consume over the day? Does this vary for you over the week usually? Or do you tend to stick to the same things over and over? Let's think about how we can add some more colour to our diet. You might simply want to make one of your changes relate to adding in ONE different colour of fruit or vegetable, after you have read the rest of this book.

It is human nature to learn about these types of polyphenols and think how amazing that is, and then think, "oh I can just get a supplement of that one!" Yes, some of these polyphenols have been studied short-term in some studies. BUT, just remember that it is likely that most of the benefit comes from:

1. Eating it WITH the fibre from the original food

2. Eating the dose that is in the original food
3. The interactions of the fibre and the polyphenol with the existing bacterial populations in the colon
4. We don't know what happens to our gut or our health if we take these for more than short- term periods. This is why I generally advise people NOT to go the supplement route.

CHAPTER 18

Is Leaky Gut Real?

A BIT MORE WATER, THE SIDE EFFECTS OF NEGLECTING PILLAR ONE AND TWO

It wasn't that long ago that leaky gut wasn't really considered something that was possible, but as science has understood more about the gut microbiome and we have better technology for assessing which compounds have passed through the intestinal barrier when they shouldn't have, that we now get a clearer picture, that yes, the gut barrier can indeed become "leaky".

When most people talk about leaky gut, they are referring to the colon being leaky.

As we learned earlier, the whole digestive tract is like an extension of the outside world. Our body does its best to protect our true internal environment, from the environment within the digestive system.

Within the colon there are thousands of species of bacteria, there are also some fungi, yeasts, phages and other viruses, plus all the bits and pieces of food particles. We don't want fragments of this stuff ending up in the bloodstream unless we specifically absorb it or tell the intestinal wall to let it through. There are some things, which the body allows to pass through the colonic cells, such as water, and things such as ions (some salts and minerals in ion form) which are allowed to pass through the existing junctions between cells.

The junctions between the cells are regulated by several proteins at different levels within the colon cells (59). Some of these proteins can now be measured in stool samples, which can give us some clues about the integrity of the gut lining. However, these are not quite tried and tested as yet, and the current (gold standard) way for testing to officially see if you have leaky gut is to consume two sugars that are non-digestible, lactulose and mannitol. Mannitol is very small and is absorbed at a pretty constant rate despite your gut barrier function, while lactulose absorption can vary because the molecule is bigger, therefore the rate of absorption into the bloodstream will depend on how "leaky" the gut environment is (59).

Unless one of my clients is having really bad and/or ongoing issues I wouldn't normally even bother testing for this because the treatment is usually along the same lines as I would give other clients regardless.

Dietary fibre is a crucial player in maintaining the integrity of the gut wall. Remember we talked about earlier how as the bacteria in our colon eat up the fibre, they produce large amounts of short-chain fatty acids? One of these acids, butyrate, is specifically beneficial for nourishing the colonic cells, and can very efficiently improve the function of the gut barrier (59).

Increasing butyrate production in the colon can be achieved by consuming more of the complex carbohydrate type starches, such as resistant starch. This is found in quite good quantities in greenish bananas, whole grain cereals (especially oats), cooked and cooled potatoes and pasta and legumes.

We also know that the other short-chain fatty acids also contribute to the health of the colon in terms of keeping those junctions nice and tight, and it is important to remember that when we eat fibre, we get a ratio of many different short-chain fatty acids produced, not just one, it's just that different fibres produce slightly different ratios, and for the resistant starches, it just leans in favour of butyrate.

To add to the complication around gut permeability, it is not just fibre that contributes to the health of the gut lining. The type and ratios of fats we consume can also have an effect. This is in addition to what we already covered when we delved into how the gut and the brain communicate, earlier.

Individuals who consume higher amounts of longer-chain unsaturated fats (EPA and DHA from fish) have a reduced incidence of ulcerative colitis, indicating that fat type might play a protective role in the colonic environment (60). We also know that the bile acids used to digest fat (some of which end up in the colon) can also regulate the permeability of the junctions between the colonic cells.

Eating a higher fat diet, means you end up with higher quantities of bile acids in your colon.

This is in part why I don't use or recommend high-fat diets (like a keto or carnivore style) because the evidence indicates that in the gut environment, it is not likely to be beneficial, especially not for the longer-term.

CHAPTER 19

Confused About Ultra-Processed Foods?

PILLAR TWO: BACTERIAL "ANTI-VITAMINS"

If you're confused about ultra-processed foods, I totally understand why.

We are bombarded with conflicting messages constantly.

On one hand, we see research and posts from our government health authorities advising us to keep our ultra-processed food consumption down and that they are bad for our health. And this is quite correct, numerous studies have now linked many poor health outcomes and weight gain with ultra-processed food consumption (61–67).

But then on the other hand, our social media feed and general advertisements keep selling us ultra-processed foods, but with a health claim on them, so they must be ok, right?

One thing I loved about nutrition when I started studying it back in the early 2000s was that it was a relatively new field as far as science goes. We are still learning and understanding what the body does with food/s, how it deals with different things in different forms and still at the infancy stage of discovering the full workings of the gut microbiome. But as we learn more and understand more, more of this work is commercialised into isolated supplements or "functional" type foods. Some of these might indeed be good for us, but how on earth is the every-day person supposed to work this out? Even with a PhD in the area, I still have to do a bit of digging when I see new things on the market, to evaluate whether they are any good.

And my second point to ponder about all of this. What is the effect on us psychologically from this constant commercialisation? The scientific innovations are fantastic, but have we really stopped to consider how this pace of marketing impacts us mentally? We have lost touch with the ability to feel confident with eating a simple diet. That's it. Our social media feeds are so full of things that can "give us a boost", "get your energy back" or "elevate your health" that we get left feeling like eating a simple diet is not enough. Not good enough. Not nutritious enough. No wonder we are tired and worn out and carrying excess weight. We need to buy that thing/supplement/food to feel better.

Food companies and supplement manufacturers are a business. The aim of the game for them is to make money and support their families. Of course they will have clever marketing and wonderful graphic design, it is part of their business. As long as we can see this for what it is and have the knowledge and confidence to decide for ourselves what our bodies need, then we can avoid getting pulled into spending money on things that 1) we don't need, 2) are not properly tested long-term, 3) are super expensive and 4) may not even help.

When it comes to actual food products, I'll delve into some of the sneaky marketing tricks a bit more below.

Okay, we've covered off why you're confused. Before we go into the details of why ultra-processed foods are not great for our gut or our health, I think it is really important to again keep in mind the big picture. No, we shouldn't be eating as much of these foods, in that they are not great for us. But should we get hung up on these foods being "bad"? NO! There are **four** pillars to gut health; If you become so extreme about avoiding these foods – then you are effectively limiting your benefits because your other pillars can't hold the table up and we are holding back our gut health from moving forward.

My focus to food, for you, is to be relaxed. Be informed. But be relaxed. For good gut health we want to bring joy to ALL the pillars.

There are three major reason why ultra-processed foods are not great for our gut (and therefore us):

1. They are missing the fibre that is/was found in the original food product.
2. They contain ingredients like preservatives, colours, emulsifiers and thickeners that can ALL disrupt the good guys in our gut.

3. They also happen to contain high amounts of simple sugars, saturated fats (or trans-fats) and/or salt. All of which can ALSO disrupt the gut microbiome.

When I first started my career as a nutritionist, I used to love doing food-additive workshops. With the power and wisdom of age and perhaps some better knowledge, these are probably the worst things to learn about. Firstly, when we delve into the world of food additives it is really complex (and quite frankly overwhelming and a little scary without a nutrition science background). Additives are used for a reason in food. They are used to make the food safe to eat or to keep it a colour or texture that the consumer will find acceptable. Many of these additives were approved for use in food well before we started researching the gut microbiome. The approvals were based on not doing harm, and not doing harm meant evaluating them for liver and/or kidney toxicity (mainly in rats or mice).

Science tells us now that many food additives can disrupt the gut microbiome. If we use a preservative in food to make it safe to eat, then the likely effect of that in the gut is that yes, it will still have that anti-bacterial effect and influence the populations of our delicate ecosystem. There's emerging evidence about emulsifiers and their potential impact on the gut too, and all of this can be a bit anxiety forming.

So, I would never run this type of workshop now. The solution is to avoid the food in the packets full stop.

If we only eat these foods occasionally as they were perhaps intended, then the risk of ongoing insults to our gut rainforest is greatly reduced. Then there's no need to stress about all the numbers. Simple.

The science of some of these individual additives is really interesting, but only If you keep your perspective and the big picture in mind. If I catch you at the supermarket thoroughly checking the labels for additive number 4567, then you'll be told to go home, make yourself a cup of tea, handed a copy of this book and made to relax for a little while.

So, if I'm telling you not to stress about ultra-processed foods, then what is the big deal then?

We know that most people are consuming upwards of 40% of their calories from these foods! It's a no-brainer then that we struggle with our weight and have chronic inflammation and issues with our gut.

There have been a few attempts to completely define what an ultra-processed food is, but the most commonly used method has been summarised for you in the image below. If a food is manufactured using ingredients that are not readily available for use at home and using methods that are generally not traditional, then it is ultra-processed. A lot of these ultra-processed foods are disguised as health products, which is probably part of the reason you've ended up here with me, because it is so confusing!

As much as I'd love to see a movement back to home cooked foods, it is really a rare thing these days with changing family dynamics, work situations and busy schedules. Despite this, we can work around it most of the time.

If I was to ask you straight out, "how much ultra-processed food do you eat?" I guarantee almost every single one of you will tell me you don't eat that much of it. Partly this is because the marketing of these foods is such that we don't consider them an ultra-processed food. They go into the records in our head as a "health food". So, give yourself a little challenge for the rest of the week. Be accountable for yourself and record everything you eat and drink for the next couple of days (as well as making a note of the calories each food provided). You'll need to be very honest with yourself and make sure you accurately record the quantities consumed and the calories they contribute.

Use the chart below to work out which of the food/s products you consumed, count as ultra-processed foods. Add up your total calories consumed and add up your calories from ultra-processed foods. Now work out as a percentage, how much of your total food intake was from ultra-processed foods? *(note: 1 calorie = 4.18 kJ, most Australian foods are listed in kJ, but some of us like to work in calories, so just make sure you record this consistently, whichever method you prefer.)*

The trick for this exercise is to be completely and utterly honest with yourself. Who is going to show up for you if you don't? Showing up for yourself starts with acknowledging where you are at.

We can't change what we don't acknowledge.

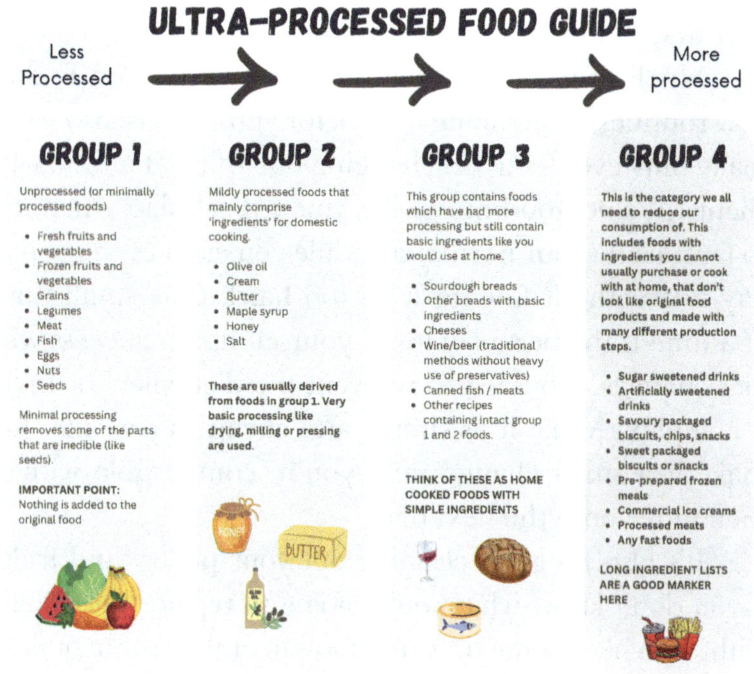

Adapted from: Crimarco A, Landry M, Gardner C. Ultra-processed Foods, Weight Gain, and Co-morbidity Risk. Curr Obes Rep. 2021 Oct 22;11:1-13.

So how do we reduce these foods in our diet, when they are everywhere?!

Were you above the 40% of calories for ultra-processed food intake? This was an Australian estimate, so I'm sure many of you are well above this figure. This is not something to beat yourself up about by the way, this is something to acknowledge is a function of the society in which we live. But, we can also acknowledge that we have a choice to do things a little better and be a better version of ourselves. Our future selves will thank us for a little extra time and thought that we put in now.

Much of the time these things are just about finding new routines and making it work for you. This is also why I really only ever focus on changing one thing at a time with clients. It's no good me giving you a meal plan when it is so far outside your normal schedule you can't even get past day two without finding it all too hard. One small thing at a time is the best way to set yourself up for success with diet changes. No need to reinvent the diet wheel or make it complex. Make it as simple and cheap as you like. Just make it a small change until you're comfortable with it, then move onto the next one.

It's also no good cleaning out your pantry and fridge if you don't know what you're going to replace these items with! You need some time and tools to embed some of these changes into your routine. Which is why I'm so big on having a one change philosophy. There's also no point me telling you something if you know it won't fit with your schedule.

"Have enough confidence with your body, your life and your intuition to know what works for you"

Some of the ultra-processed foods will disappear on their own as you add in more fruits and vegetables each week. Remember we want to keep the focus on ADDING things that are more healthful, and not focusing on restricting or depriving ourselves.

So, this chapter of the book is towards the end for a reason. Focus on the positive aspects of adding in one extra fruit or veg or whole grain each week for at least the first month or two. You might find that by doing this you automatically reduced your consumption of ultra-processed foods without even thinking about it consciously. This is absolutely perfect! Progress without is guilt is 100% the right approach.

If you feel like you've still got a bit of work to do on your ultra-processed food consumption, then some of my top suggestions are listed below.

1. This might be a bit obvious but sometimes spelling out the obvious is quite necessary. Don't have them in the house. It forces you to think of something else to eat if you are indeed really hungry. If you really NEED it and have to go to the shops to buy it, then likely 90% of the time you won't be bothered. Mission accomplished!
2. Yoghurt is a great source of calcium, protein and probiotics. But the flavoured ones are full of sugar, artificial sweeteners or other thickeners we don't need. The best ones are the plain and unsweetened Greek yoghurts. These are often cheaper too which is a double bonus. Depending on what flavour mood you are in you can add your own flavour. Honey, berries, cocoa + a little bit of

sugar, banana, etc. you get the idea. Doesn't take more than 1 min of extra prep time.

3. Dried fruits are great for the sweet cravings after dinner. A couple of prunes also have great amounts of polyphenols (obviously choose the ones that work best for you), and if you can find preservative free ones, even better.
4. Plain popcorn is fantastic to get the salty cravings, while actually counting as a whole grain serve in one go (without the butter obviously).
5. Instead of muesli bars or processed bars in packets, a little container of nuts is a very quick and easy alternative. Just remember 6-8 nuts counts as 1 serve.
6. Bake a batch of something that your family likes, cut it up and put it in the freezer on the weekend. Banana bread is a great way to use up the old bananas in the fruit bowl. I always add extra seeds/grains, use wholemeal flour and add dates or other dried fruits too, whatever works for your family and tastes. Have the confidence to change a recipe. It's actually harder than you think to stuff up in the kitchen.
7. If you drink plant-based milks, find one with the smallest list of ingredients.
8. A piece of toast or a bowl of oats is a perfectly acceptable snack. Bonus points if it is grainy bread.

9. Opt for quality over quantity. Opting for a premium version of whatever you were looking for, such as ice cream, might mean you get a more traditionally made version, which is richer, less processed and tastes pretty darn nice. So, taking this option means you can enjoy feeling like a true foodie, but it's expensive and rich enough we usually eat way less of it. Same goes for dark chocolate.

WHAT ABOUT SUGAR?

One of the most important food components I want to delve into for this chapter is the effect of simple sugars on our gut microbiome.

We all know that excess sugars in general are not good for us and that they are associated with things like diabetes. But did you know that they can also change our gut microbiome composition (44,45,68)?

As I mentioned before, I was taught that all of our macronutrients were absorbed in the small intestine. We now know that this process is indeed not 100% efficient at all! In fact, eating too much of anything all in one go, will limit the amount that we can absorb. This is simply because there isn't enough time to absorb it all before it moves on and through to the colon. Or we exceed the capacity of the little transporters that take it out of the mixture and into our bloodstream. Either way, there's too much for the small intestine to cope with and it ends up in the colon.

The bacteria in the colon have a party when they get hit with simple sugars. Because these are readily digestible and they have bonds which many more species have the ability to utilise, we see increases in species that can use these up quickly. These species are also the ones that have the ability degrade our protective mucus layer and increase permeability and inflammation (44,45,68).

So, if you get a funny stomach after eating a lot of sweets in one go, this is what is happening. In isolation or just in once off scenarios this is manageable. The problem is that when we continually feed these bacteria the simple sugars, they continue to degrade the mucus layer (44,45,68) and trigger inflammation. Simply cutting back simple sugar intake and increasing your fibre intake is THE perfect way to improve your gut and overall health.

The simple sugars we are talking about here:

1. Anything with high added sugars (falls into ultra-processed food category anyway). Things like high-fructose corn syrup, invert syrup, juice concentrates all count as added sugars.
2. High amounts of table sugar in one go, such as lollies or sweets (these can also count as an ultra-processed food.)

Remember not to confuse the sugars found in WHOLE fruits as falling into this category. Yes, they have simple sugars. But they are bound up with fibre and polyphenols and in much smaller quantities than we find in ultra-processed foods. I've talked to many people who say they don't eat fruit because...*sugar*... but then eat stuff in packets instead... This is the wrong approach!

If you've read this chapter and are inspired to clean out your whole pantry over the weekend, just remember the power of the small changes. They are achievable. They add up. They are easy.

We want this transformation to be easy. That is the point of the whole thing. Do it with ease! And joy! And fun!

CHAPTER 20

Bacteria Can Get Hangovers Too

PILLAR THREE: LIFESTYLE FACTORS

Often when we talk about diets and gut health, people talk about adding supplements in and changing diets, but we forget to mention that alcohol can play a big part in the health of our gut environment.

When the Mediterranean diet was first documented in the scientific literature, it was thought that the benefit for this diet was due to the olive oil and the red wine. Overly simplistic, yes, but that was the thinking at the time.

We now know a little bit more and perhaps have the benefit of a bit of hindsight. Yes, the extra virgin olive oil is a big contributing factor to the success of the Mediterranean diet. But the red wine?

Research now shows us quite clearly that alcohol is pretty toxic to most tissues in the body (we did know this before, but perhaps scientists were hopeful for the red wine?). After we consume it, it is rapidly absorbed into our bloodstream and turned into acetaldehyde. Both alcohol (ethanol) and acetaldehyde can have detrimental effects on our whole body. In the gut, it can increase the gaps in between cells, leading to a temporary state of leaky gut, which has a downstream effect of causing some inflammation. It also reduces the production of the beneficial short-chain fatty acids by the microbiome, which further exacerbates these effects. Every 10 g increase in alcohol consumption is associated with 1.07 x the risk of colorectal cancer (69).

The reason that the red wine portion of the Mediterranean diet was thought to be protective, was because of the polyphenols from the grapes. Perhaps this possibly offset the effect of the alcohol. There is evidence that the resveratrol, from the red grapes, can be protective in the gut environment, and can help prevent the conversion of a metabolite known to impact cardiovascular disease (called TMAO) (70,71). This might be one of those polyphenols that is better utilised as a pharmacological treatment in at-risk patients, because telling patients with cardiovascular disease to drink wine for the polyphenols is not good medical advice! There are other foods which contain resveratrol, like eating the red grapes. Berries and peanuts also contain this compound, but not in the quantities we see in red wine.

At this stage, there is still not clear evidence for long-term use of these compounds as supplements, as we have talked about before. But back to the alcohol story. Long-term, alcohol does not have good support behind its consumption, especially when it comes to gut health.

Short- term, we all know it doesn't make us feel good the next day. It effects our sleep quality, our hydration status, our mental alertness and our food intake. If you have any sort of fitness tracker watch or Oura ring, you might have already noticed that one or two drinks is enough to muck up all the metrics overnight, especially your heart rate variability, which is used to measure stress. If you want to cut down your drinking, then I highly recommend getting a fitness watch or ring that tracks heart rate variability and has advanced sleep tracking. Compare your sleep and your heart rate variability between the days you don't have anything to drink, with the days you do. This is enough wow all by itself to help you decide if you want to have a drink or not.

The take home-message is that alcohol in all doses is not helpful and in fact harmful for most of our cells in our body.

The red part of red wine is the only beneficial component in there, but this can be found in other foods too, so let's focus on those rather than drinking the wine. As we get older, we often have less time and patience for feeling off the day after having a few drinks.

Go back to the mind map from earlier, look at what you wrote down about how you want to show up in this world. Does your usual alcohol consumption support those things? If the answer is no, then think about how you can still be social and fun and happy without the drinking.

But, also keep in mind the big picture. Yes, alcohol is not great for most of our organ systems. Yes, it mucks up our sleep and our mood and our eating patterns. But is it also worth stressing about now and again if we go out for dinner with friends? Occasional consumption in the context of your whole life needs to be weighed up. This whole book is about empowering yourself to make informed and relaxed decisions. So read the info, know the info and then decide if you want to have a drink or not. And then don't stress about your decision.

CHAPTER 21

Bacteria Love a Bit of Exercise

PILLAR THREE: LIFESTYLE FACTORS

It is pretty amazing to think that exercise can even remotely influence the bacterial population in the colon – because we are not changing the food supply we are providing it.

But let's think about what does change when we do some exercise. Our muscles, when they are exercising release metabolites into the blood stream (72,73), which can change the way we take up and utilise glucose and amino acids from the blood. There are changes in the blood supply and metabolites in the colon. We also get changes in actual blood flow happening too because when we exercise, blood gets diverted AWAY from our digestive tract and to the muscles that need it.

It is really interesting that these changes and the bit of stress that exercise puts on the digestive system, improves its overall function. Much like anything with our body, a little bit of stress makes things more efficient. Like doing weights, putting a bit of stress on your muscles, forces them to grow and become stronger. Doing exercise forces your cardiovascular system to become stronger, practising cold exposure forces your body to become more efficient at warming itself up.

Studies of endurance athletes show they have greater abundances of beneficial bacterial species, greater overall diversity and reduced low-grade inflammation, than non-athletes (72). In animal studies, we also see increases in the bacteria known to be beneficial during exercise, along with increases in the super beneficial short-chain fatty acids (butyrate in particular), which supports many of the health benefits associated with exercise in the first place. A human study examining people of different levels of fitness, but with similar diets, also supports this finding (74).

The difficult thing about studying this in every-day people is that microbiome diversity is also linked with body fat percentage, so any sort of exercise we do also usually reduces our body fat. So are the changes in microbiome due to the change in body fat or a direct result of the exercise? (75)

The message so far is that exercise can improve our gut microbiome diversity (so the number of species living in there and how they are distributed) and it can also increase the rate of production of the beneficial short-chain fatty acids. In particular, butyrate.

Now the really interesting and very important linking point here is that this increase in short-chain fatty acid production is also linked with better brain health (73), which reduces our risk for things like anxiety and depression and has overall effect of improving mood. So, overall, more evidence that every system in the body is linked.

This is why this book is focused on ALL these areas. Because we can't have one without the other. We can increase our short-chain fatty acid production with diet, but we can also increase it with exercise, both of which can help us feel awesome, and then we feel like doing more. It's a circle of benefits supporting more benefits.

You might be thinking well what sort of exercise is best? Much of the research to date on the gut microbiome and exercise has only been done in athletes, so my answer to that is that it doesn't matter as long as you do something! Doing something is better than doing nothing. If you tell me you either don't like exercise or you can't fit it in to their day, then you need to find some form of exercise that brings you joy.

You need to make it a priority to fit it into your day. It is always easier to get it done earlier in the day before it becomes easy for things to get busy, kids to get crazy or the tiredness sets in. It's about choosing yourself.

Some influencers are pretty outspoken about calling you out for the time you might waste on social media or similar, and yes, I do think we can utilise some of that time better, but don't get to the point where you feel guilty for not giving yourself any down time either. Life has to be a balance. You need to be tough and show up for yourself sometimes, but you also need to be kind to yourself and nurture yourself with some rest or a nap under the doona sometimes too.

You need to work out your own limits for when you can push yourself and when you should take it easy. And even though I'm nearly 48 I still have to learn my lessons for this, usually by making a mistake of doing too much, then feeling terrible for a day or two afterwards. It's about learning, really learning, to what our body is telling us. It would be great to have consistent sleep and consistent energy every day and to know how much we can plan to do on any given day. Our body just doesn't work to this level of machine status. There are ebbs and flows with our sleep, with our energy, with our tiredness and some of it is not even logical to try and work out why it is different from day to day. It just is. Tune in and listen.

If you haven't exercised for a while, then it might be hard at first to work out if that exercise is actually going to bring you joy because that part where your fitness is increasing might feel a bit hard for a week or two. My advice here is to try each type of exercise for at least 3-4 weeks before you make a decision on whether it is something you want to stick at or not.

I've always been pretty fit, but never ran that much (I always preferred swimming). Enough to get by, but never a runner. I decided a couple of years ago I was going to enter a half-marathon. Trained for two months, did the half marathon and still didn't feel like I really got the running thing. I just stuck at it for some reason, I don't really know why, it was just something I wanted to get better at. So, over the past few years, I've kept running a few times a week. It's actually only now that I really and truly love it. I'm still not fast or good at it, but I love it. It brings me so much joy to get out in the fresh air with the music on and feel so free, so that is really all that matters.

This is just a reminder that exercise doesn't have to be something you're good at. You can pretty well suck at it actually, but if you're moving, you're ahead of most people and for that you need to give yourself a pat on the back. If you're new to exercising then doing this process with a friend or enrolling in a Zumba class together, the joy can come from laughing with and at each other. More joy comes from feeling good afterwards, from feeling strong, from feeling fit and sleeping better because you got out and did something.

Now similar to my one change philosophy, I have similar philosophy for exercise. You can't and won't sustain ANY changes to your exercise routine if you try and do too much all at once before you've embedded the changes in your lifestyle. So, telling yourself you're going to start running and you're going to do an hour a day every day is just setting yourself up for failure because by Day 2 your body is totally exhausted and you can't continue the week.

How to get started then if you're not sure what exercise to start with? Think about when it is you're at your most happy. Is it being outside? Is it dancing? Is it music? Start with that. Whatever your answer is there, think about some kind of exercise that you can combine with this.

Now think about your schedule and your priorities.

If you choose to put YOU at the top of your priority list, what can you fit in this week? If you schedule it into your calendar, it is more likely to get done. If you commit to doing something with a friend, it is more likely to get done. We just want to start being a little more active. By not doing too much too soon, by doing something fun and doing something that you know is going to make you feel good. As you start to feel better with your diet changes you might actually surprise yourself and be able to add more things in each week.

Remember going from zero to hero with exercise is only setting yourself up for failure.

And doing something small is better than doing nothing.

CHAPTER 22

Your Gut Bacteria and Your Bones are Friends

THE AMAZING LINKS BETWEEN THE PILLARS

The simple fact that your bone health is even remotely linked to your gut microbiome is the most mind-blowing thing ever. This is why I love science and why I keep telling people about how amazing the human body is. It is also yet another example of the intricate and complex web of linking between that rainforest in your gut and the rest of your body.

There is now a good body of literature supporting this gut-bone-axis (76–79) and, in particular, for middle-aged women, having a healthy gut ecosystem can really change the game for keeping your bones strong as you age.

How does this work though? How can our gut bacteria possibly influence the health of our bones?

You might think about your bones as a solid, static scaffold for the rest of your body. However, your bones are constantly in a state of remodelling. They are like a house constantly under renovation. There is bone breakdown and bone building occurring constantly. So over time, if our rate of breakdown is greater than our building phase, we can end up with osteopenia or osteoporosis.

As we get a bit older, it takes a bit more effort to keep your body focused on not giving up on the building works, when it comes to your bones. Your body is in fact still a teenager at heart, it really can't be bothered keeping things maintained, unless is really, really has to. We have to keep telling our body that yes, our bones are in fact required, so please keep them strong. We do this by doing some weight bearing exercise (and also by keeping our nutrition adequate). This places a little bit of stress on the bones and gives the 'Hello, yes, I am required signal' to our bone builders.

When it comes to bone breakdown, this is the part of the equation that seems to be linked to the gut microbiome. The first is via the anti-inflammatory effect of short-chain fatty acids produced when gut bacteria consume (or ferment) plant fibres. These short-chain fatty acids are proposed to have several benefits when it comes to your bones. The reduction in inflammatory markers from short chain fatty acid production, down regulates the bone breakdown pathways. The fact that these little fatty acids are in fact acidic, helps to acidify the colon. This has the effect of ionising any remaining calcium in the colon and therefore helps it be absorbed. In addition, short chain fatty acid production also seems to benefit bacterial production of vitamin B12 and K, both of which are important for healthy metabolic function. Finally, the short-chain fatty acids may also stimulate the production of receptors for vitamin D, also required for healthy bones (80).

All of these proposed mechanisms rely on sufficient short-chain fatty acid production in a very complex but beautiful cascade of benefits. Which really tells the story that we need sufficient (or perhaps more) fibre than we might have paid attention to before, in order to help our bones stay strong as we get older.

This of course, is in addition to eating sufficient calcium and protein too ☺. [it is complex isn't it?]

While a lot of this mechanistic scientific investigation has been done in mice or rats, we've seen a few human studies where increased fibre has been studied from specific food sources to examine the effect on bone mineral density. Giving post-menopausal women 50g of prunes each day (this equates to about 5-6 prunes) over 12 months (81,82) resulted in a greater than 1% improvement in bone mineral density (this sounds small but can be quite significant, because we aren't talking about any further losses here, but gains). Interestingly, the women who saw the biggest benefit hosted specific bacterial genera linked with bone health (83). The authors of these studies hypothesise it is the interaction between the fibre and polyphenols in the prune and the bacteria, which lead to the slowing down or inhibition of the bone breakdown process.

I really love studies which first, use whole foods. Prunes have also been consumed as part of dietary patterns over a very long period of time, so we know they have a good track record of safety for long term use. They are also cheap and very tasty!

However, fibre isn't the only part of the story for bone health though, because we know that vegans and vegetarians traditionally eat more fibre than omnivores, however, epidemiological evidence shows that while this group has lower risk of many chronic disease outcomes, they also have lower bone mineral density (84). This may be due to many things, including lower calcium intake (via the exclusion of dairy), lower overall protein intake and lower intake of other nutrients like vitamin B12. My take home message here is that if you are vegan or vegetarian for whatever reason, then it is important to get some professional advice here sooner rather than later, so we can protect your precious bones. The traditional recommendations for adequate protein intake may not be sufficient for optimal health, including that of our bones, we will delve into this more in the next chapter.

CHAPTER 23

Protein is Complicated

THE AMAZING LINKS BETWEEN THE PILLARS

At the time of writing this book, the whole protein message has been lapped up by supplement companies and food companies alike. Everything has a protein claim on it. It's the '99% fat free' of the 2020s. I dismissed most of this in the early few years of this as just marketing, but more and more research has suggested our human body works better with a little more protein than perhaps we first considered. Most RDI's are set for protein intake at around 0.84g/kg for men and 0.75g/kg for women (85), but this is one of those cases where avoiding deficiency is quite different from optimal function.

There is solid evidence now to suggest intakes of around 1.2 g/kg should be the minimum (86). If you are female entering perimenopause, doing any sort of weight training or regular physical activity, then intakes a little higher than this, might be best. For example, a person weighing 70kg, this takes your target from 56g to somewhere between 84 and 112g (1.6 g/kg). There is actually a big difference between these two intakes in terms of actual food. Especially if we also need to eat the required number of calories, fibre and other nutrients that are also important.

I suggested earlier in the book it is a good idea to hold yourself accountable to make sure you are hitting your fibre targets, but it is also important to do this for protein. If you're female, you should also check you are meeting your calcium and iron requirements too.

The complicating thing about eating protein is that it isn't always desirable in the gut microbiome environment. Protein breakdown in the colon produces waste that can be toxic to the cells of the colon (such phenols, cresols and ammonia) (37–39). And the type of bacteria that eat up the leftover proteins are not necessarily any of the good guys. But, you need to weigh this up for yourself – if you get really smelly gas, then there's probably too much protein fermentation happening, increasing your fibre intake might help balance this out.

This is also why it is a good idea to space out your intake through the day. If you are exercising, then having some sort of meal with protein after exercise and eating sufficient calories and carbohydrates (and fibre) ensures that the protein can do its job and get to where it needs to be used for muscles and bones and other important cellular processes (87).

We also need to consider the quality of the protein we are eating. Red and processed meats have good evidence supporting links with colorectal cancer, diabetes and heart disease (88–90), so I usually recommend people stick to eating protein from plants first, then things like dairy/yoghurt/whey protein, then fish, chicken or eggs, before delving into the red meat category.

It's also a good idea to not chug your protein smoothies too fast. There is very little research in the area of protein shakes and the gut microbiome, but human physiology applies here very sensibly. We want to maximise the amount of protein we absorb in the small intestine and not end up with too much of it in the colon, so keep this in mind before you drink the whole lot in 30 seconds flat. While protein powders can be highly processed, if you find a plain, unflavoured or unsweetened one, these can be a good addition to your day to ensure you are getting your protein requirements met. A mixed plant protein or unflavoured whey would be my go-to for recommendations here.

But track and try to hit your target intake from actual food and your real diet first. Protein powders are also very expensive, so if you can hit your targets from food and still meet your fibre goals, then that is fantastic. We just don't want to prioritise protein in place of fibre, because this puts our gut at a complete disadvantage. The protein to fibre ratio can help dilute some of the more toxic protein metabolites in the colon. The two must go hand in hand.

Oh, and remember earlier we mentioned how we have to disassemble the proteins into amino acids in order to absorb them? They don't magically get reassembled back to muscle cells unless we are using them. That's an important point to remember!

CHAPTER 24

Avoiding Label Stress

WATERING YOUR GARDEN

I'm beginning this chapter with a bit of a caveat. I am going to walk you through nutrition labels, but I do NOT want you spending 30 minutes checking every ingredient in great detail while you are doing your shopping.

Your main goal is to eat less (way less) of the things in packets. So, for the few items that fall into this category, I want you to really think through whether it is worth all the stress to worry so much about these?

Keep the big picture in mind. This is important. There is absolutely no point doing all this work on your mindset, doing exercise and eating more fibre if you anxiously stress about all the little ingredients when you do your shopping. Remember stress has a big role in our gut health. Don't underestimate this and get caught up on the little things. It is the big picture that matters.

Now that we have that straight, we are going get straight into those nutrition labels.

We're going over an Australian version, well because I'm Aussie and this is where most of my clients live.

These are my top six things to check, and we will go through each of them in a bit more detail.

1. Serving size.
2. Ingredient list. Look at the length.
3. Fibre content. Did they add fibre/s?
4. Sugar content. Is it added or natural?
5. Fat. Check for saturated fats.
6. Allergens.

CALORIES VS KILOJOULES

Before we start with my list, we do need to clarify the difference between calories and kilojoules. Calories are imperial way of measuring energy, which is used in the United States, while Australia uses the metric measurement of kilojoules. 1 calorie = 4.18 kilojoules. Australian food panels have kilojoules.

The first part of tricky marketing by food companies starts with the serving size.

SERVING SIZE

They might make a claim that there's only x grams of sugar per serve on the front. But when you turn it over and check the back, we can see that a serve size is only half of the packet. When really you would (and most people would) eat the whole thing in one go.

Before we even check ANY of the ingredients, it's already a bit misleading. So, the very first thing we should do is have a think about how much of this packet of whatever we are likely to eat? Is it the whole thing? Or just half? Or is the serve size accurate for you?

The chocolate bars where there are two sections inside the packet are a good example of this. The back says there's two serves in there. I don't know about you, but If I'm choosing chocolate, I'm eating the whole thing.

The food companies unfortunately rely on us not thinking very hard when we make these purchases, because hey, we already purchased it based on that front label, so they already won!

THE INGREDIENT LIST

Tip number 2 is the ingredient list. This is how we can work out if the food is firstly ultra-processed or not, and two – if it is so long and confusing, then we need to ask ourselves do we really need this? If there are more than around five ingredients on the panel, then it likely is an ultra-processed food (but there can be some nuances here).

Simple foods usually have simple ingredients. Like a sourdough bread, with the ingredients:

WHEAT FLOUR, WATER, SUGAR, SALT, CULTURE

Compared to an ultra-processed bread with the following list:

Unbleached **Wheat** Flour, Water, **Wheat** Fibre, Modified Tapioca Starch (1412), Baker's Yeast, Vinegar, **Wheat** Gluten,

Iodised Salt, Vegetable Gum (412), Canola Oil, **Soy** Flour, Vegetable Emulsifiers (481, 472e, 471), Minerals (Iron, Zinc), Vitamins (Vitamin E, Niacin, Thiamin, Vitamin B6, Folic Acid), Processing Aid (**Wheat**).

The simpler and the smaller the ingredient list, the better. But again, I need to stress, you need to think about how much of this food you are going to eat or what the role of it is in your diet. If it is a small, sometimes type thing, then really, it's not worth stressing about too much. But if it something like bread, you eat multiple times per day, then yes, a good idea to find an option which is less processed.

FIBRE CONTENT

Now we are tracking back to our friend called fibre. Just to recap, it is one term but a large and very diverse group of compounds with the main definition of resisting digestion in the small intestine and providing food for microbes in the large intestine.

We've also looked at our own diet and the sources of fibre and where it is coming from.

After looking at the ingredient list, checking the fibre content is a good place to start, because it gives us an idea of two things:

1. how much of the original plant food might be left in the product
2. or whether there are other ingredients which provide the fibre

When we talk about fibre, we are talking about it in terms of grams / 100 g. Not per serve. There is a difference because a serve size could be all different things. The 100 g column is the last column on the nutrition panel.

Fibre content per 100 g: When looking at nutrition labels, a good rule of thumb is:

- Low fibre: Less than 3 g per 100 g
- Good source of fibre: 3-6 g per 100 g
- High fibre: More than 6 g per 100 g

Serving size consideration: While we often look at per 100 g values, it's crucial to consider the typical serving size of the food. Some foods may have a high fibre content per 100 g, but if the serving size is small, the actual fibre intake might be less significant.

Now I want you to also think about the fibre content I just mentioned because it applies really well to packet foods, which don't usually have high amounts of water in them. Think breads, pastas, cereals, etc.

WHAT ABOUT AN APPLE?

An apple contains around 2.4 g fibre per 100 g. So an average apple which weighs 150 g would have 3.6 g fibre. Because we would usually eat the whole apple right?

BUT

This is where we need to put things in perspective. Because an apple contains around or just less than 90%

water. So that 2.4 grams of fibre is contained in only about 10 grams of apple if we compare the dry weights.

The take home message is that whole foods, fruits and vegetables contain a lot of water, so their bang for their buck in terms of fibre content is really high.

This is why you can't really compare dry packet foods with a fibre content on the nutrition label with fresh foods, because you might come back and tell me that this packet food you found has way more fibre than an apple.

This guide is really useful for packet foods, but remember that ANY fruit or vegetable is good for you in terms of fibre, plus it has all the polyphenols and other beneficial compounds. Variety of fibre is key here.

The other thing to consider with fibre and packet foods is the source of the fibre. Have they added something to make it have that fibre content or does it come from the food itself.

These isolated fibres ADDED to foods might be quite good for your gut. But they could equally cause you pain, gas or bloating or all of the above. So if you do get symptoms after eating a so called gut friendly ultra-processed food, then write down what the food was and the ingredients and then you can chat with your health professional (obviously one that is well educated on the gut) about that particular fibre.

SWEET TRICKS

Now we've talked about fibre, let's talk about sugar.

Simple sugars are not great for our gut bacteria. The types of bacteria these support are some good ones, but also some not great ones. These are some of the species that can degrade our protective mucus layer, so keeping the simple sugars low is a good idea. And I don't mean from fruit, remember the sugars in fruit are pre-wrapped in fibre and polyphenols, so these are not the ones that cause us harm.

The sugars I am talking about are the ones in ultra-processed foods, mainly because the quantities in these foods are high and they can seem very hidden, even in foods which say they have no added sugar.

Manufacturers are and have been really clever at how they label and market these foods, because they know they can claim they haven't added actual sugar. But what they have added instead is fruit juice concentrate, which is.. yes, you guessed it, basically a sugar syrup. And if they used a fruit juice concentrate which had fibre or polyphenols in it, we might have to think a bit about it, but the most common one used in ultra-processed foods is pear juice. Because it is mildly flavoured, mildly coloured and nice and sweet (and cheap).

In Australia, we've had a bit of conversation about regulation of added sugars and nutrition labels for a while. It hasn't yet been successful, but what nutrition professionals have been asking for is that manufacturers are required to list on the nutrition panel, what is natural sugar (from the food) and what is added sugar. Even so, where would we stand with pear juice concentrate? It might still be grey because manufacturers claim that the sugar is from the pears, not because they added pear juice concentrate to have a clean label (but in fact they added it because it acted as a sweetener).

As with most nutrition concepts there are plenty of exceptions. In your head right now you might be asking, well what about artificial sweeteners? These were so popular when they were first developed and launched, but as we start to learn more about how they are metabolised and interact with the gut microbiome, my message is to avoid them where possible. If you want something sweet, have the REAL thing, have less of it, and then have it less often.

Feeling the complexity and confusion here? Yes, me too, and this is one of the reasons that people end up here, because they are confused. So, this is why it is so important to keep that big picture in your mind because this helps you keep all these nuances in perspective.

FATS

Adding fat to foods is not new. Cooking with fat, carbohydrates and either salt or sugar is the ultimate taste sensation and really hits all of our instinctive spots on our palate.

Have you tried dry roasting potatoes without any oil? I do this occasionally and they are nice, but nowhere near as good as when they have some salt and extra virgin olive oil added first.

Now remember, fat is 100% calories. It is 100% fat. So, if you ever see something labelled as lite olive oil, then they are referring to the colour or the flavour, not the calories (again a tricky tactic).

We've also talking previously about how extra virgin olive oil is good for us. This is true. The problem with UPFs is that extra virgin olive oil is expensive. Even foods like tuna which claim to be packed in olive oil, you might find has an asterisk next to it with a little tiny note at the bottom, saying "olive oil BLEND" which means it might only contain 10% olive oil and 90% other cheap oils. Plant and seed oils are not harmful for us, but I'm just pointing out that it's not always what we thought it was.

Food manufacturers' aim is to make a profit right?

They find a cheaper oil to use.

And these cheaper oils can be high in saturated fats (which can be inflammatory [most plant-based oils or seed oils are NOT harmful]); or highly processed fats that end up being hydrogenated (also inflammatory).

I've got nothing against having added fats, but the fats are not the sort that we need to be eating and completely not the sort we thought we were actually buying when we saw the 'olive oil*' on the label.

This is just another reason why sticking to actual food is WAY easier, because we don't even need to think about all these fine print issues or have a degree in Nutrition just to interpret the label.

Continuing to cut down your ultra-processed food consumption is a good idea, because I could spend two hours talking to you about all the different issues with different ultra-processed foods. For example, low fat foods like mayonnaise might not contain as much in the way of oils, but to retain the texture, they contain more sugar and thickeners.

The things to look out for or just to be aware of, are:

- Low fat foods are likely contain added salts, sugars, thickeners, other preservatives, etc.
- Olive oil might be labelled as an olive oil blend, which might mean there is not much extra virgin olive oil in there at all.

Any oil is not a low-calorie food, so if it is labelled as 'lite', then it is referring to the colour or flavour.

Saturated fats and trans fats are the ones we want to reduce.

BUT cutting out the UPFs is easier than trying to swap them with something, because other similar foods are also going to have detrimental properties to them.

ALLERGENS

The last of my top shopping tips are the allergens. Anyone here who has an allergy will be so on top of this, but if you buy anything in a packet in Australia, it is required to have an allergen statement. On the ingredient list, you will also notice that anything that is classed as an allergen is in bold.

You can also be absolutely allergic to something that doesn't fall onto this list!

But the common ones (that are marked in bold on an ingredient list) are: wheat, fish, crustacean, mollusc, egg, milk, lupin, peanut, soy, soya, soybean, sesame, almond, Brazil nut, cashew, hazelnut, macadamia, pecan, pistachio, pine nut, walnut, barley, oats, rye and sulphites (FSANZ).

An allergy is very different from being a bit intolerant to something. Being a bit intolerant means, we might get some uncomfortable symptoms when we eat that food, but we will be okay within a short amount of time.

An allergy, however, is an immediate, immune response to the attacking food. The body thinks it is under attack, so it mounts this huge immune response to try and help, but in fact, this can be deadly. Even in molecular quantities. Eaten peanut butter? Don't go anywhere near your friend who is deathly allergic to peanuts. Wash your hands, brush your teeth first. Anyone with an allergy is very vigilant checking ingredients, to make sure they don't accidentally consume something they can't eat.

Allergies have been on the increase in Western society over the last 20 years, so I am sure we all know someone close to us who lives with this fear every day. There is a lot of research in this area at the moment and I am quietly confident science will develop a cure for this in our lifetimes, and it will likely have something to do with the gut microbiome!

CHAPTER 25

What About Supplements?

WATERING YOUR GARDEN

When the recommended dietary intakes were released in Australia, the purpose of them was to provide some guidance to the population on sufficient nutrient intake to avoid deficiency syndromes (91).

Scientists estimate the average requirement for a population and set a safety factor in there, to ensure that the amount recommended meets the needs of most of the population (97.5% to be exact, two standard deviations if you like a bit of maths).

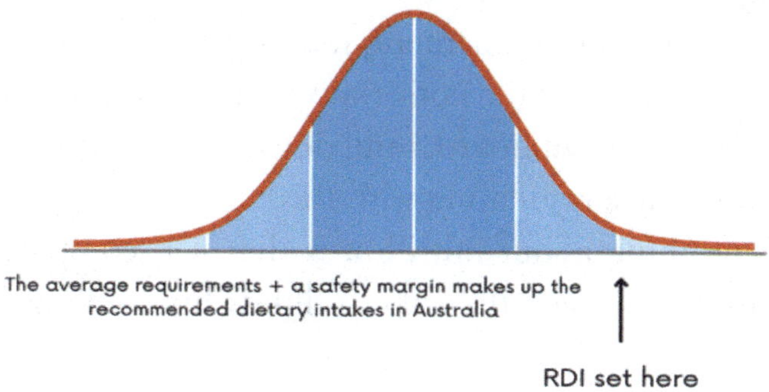

The thing about health is that deficiency syndromes and optimal functioning for health can be different scenarios. We might need a certain amount of a particular nutrient, like Vitamin C for example, to avoid a deficiency disease like scurvy. (The Australian RDI is 45 mg/day for adults)(92) and we also know we exceed our absorptive capacity of the intestines at around 1000mg/day, so the actual amount required individually for optimal function and absorption might be somewhere in the middle. This discrepancy between avoiding deficiency and optimal function is where things go a little astray. As humans we have this inbuilt functioning that says, 'well if that is good for us, then more must be even better!'.

The supplement industry has really capitalised on our thinking around this. Put something in a bottle, give it some fancy clean label and some ads about how it will fix your everything problem and bingo, we lap it all up and the company selling it makes astronomical profits. The thing is, we kind of know in our heart already, that type of quick fix is unlikely to work. But the messaging on the ads or testimonial can be so convincing that we are simply just willing to give it a shot. I know in the past when I've caved and bought some supplement, that it gets taken for a week or two, then we don't notice anything, so the rest of the bottle sits in the cupboard, until one day it gets thrown out. I know you are resonating with this…

The thing about nutrition is that it is complex. It is a lot more complex than the wellness huns selling MLM supplements understand. More definitely does not equal better. More can equal better up to a point, but more can also be toxic at the right dose. Even for water.

One of my biggest philosophies across all my platforms is that marketing and profit has taken over health. We are bombarded with this constant fear of "not having enough", "not being well enough", "not eating properly", "our food just doesn't have nutrition anymore". Just this constant feeling being portrayed to us that we are not enough.

We have the power to jump right off this wagon.

We are, and you are, enough.

If you live in a Western society (i.e. a wealthy society like ours), eat some fruit and vegetables (which I am assuming you do because you are here) then you don't need 99% of the supplements on the market.

I reserved 1% there for women who are low on iron, for vegans and vegetarians who need the b12 and post-menopausal women who might benefit from calcium + vitamin D. That 1% becomes more of a pharmaceutical need than a want to satisfy the not enough-ness.

There is slightly more regulation in Australia for supplements than there is in the United States, but we need to be quite wary here.

- Does the product even contain what it says it has in it? (some smaller studies indicate via testing that this might be a bigger issue than previously thought) (93).

- How does the product interact with the gut microbiome? For 99% of these, we don't know.
- What happens to our bodies when we take them for 1+ years? Again for 99% of these, we don't know.
- What claim are they making? Claims are very well regulated here, so it should either say "traditionally used for" or have no claim. However, if you've purchased something online from overseas, it might have all sorts of claims on it, that may or may not have any basis to them.
- They are expensive! You may have easily spent more on supplements in the last month than you have on this book. Structuring your diet and lifestyle based on the four pillars of gut health, really eliminates your need for any supplement at all (except for my 1% who need them for a medical reason).

If you do ever need a supplement - my advice is to only ever get exactly the one your health professional prescribes, or if you are buying it yourself, don't get caught up thinking the one with all the other added things is better. The plain ones giving you just what you need are the good ones.

CHAPTER 26

What About Probiotics?

WATERING YOUR GARDEN

This is a super complex area.

It's not just as straightforward as going to the local pharmacy and buying a bottle of whatever they recommend.

Remember earlier I talked about how our gut microbiome is like a rainforest?

Taking a probiotic is like introducing a new species to the forest. Will it be able to grow? Has it got enough food? Is it the right species to be able to thrive here? Is it going to cause other species to be affected?

Lots of questions and only some answers here.

Probiotics also fall into the category of big business. With the research in this area, with new technologies emerging, there has been an explosion of new products on the market. Some of these only have sketchy clinical studies to support their claims with very few participants, or in very specific clinical conditions.

Do you remember when you used to go to the pharmacy to buy a probiotic and you had to go to the fridge to get them? It is super cool that we don't have to do this now because scientists worked out we could freeze dry them and they would come alive again when they were exposed to moisture.

The issue with the number of new products on the market and all the different types is that it is really difficult for us as consumers to evaluate what we actually might need, or how strong the evidence is supporting its use. The other issue with going to the pharmacy is that the pharmacist or the assistant is likely relying on information given to them by the actual manufacturer of the product, which removes their ability to think critically about the use of it in the first place. The product also might benefit one person but make another feel worse.

In research to make clinical recommendations, we pool a large number of studies all together and see, across all of the studies (accounting for the study participant differences etc.) what the effect is. This is called a meta-analysis. The problem with doing a meta-analysis for probiotic use is that there are thousands of different bacterial species and strains that might have been used in those clinical studies. So, we should be evaluating them separately or at least be quite specific when we group them together to work out if we should recommend them or not.

I'm in a large number of online forums about gut health, and I often see people reporting side effects, and not necessarily nice ones, from taking a probiotic and they are not sure whether they should continue taking it or not, because they have a perception that they are only beneficial and they could not possibly cause harm.

My advice for probiotics is to tread carefully. There is some good evidence for some conditions, for some species/strains of bacteria. But this should really be advice that is given to you individually specific for your condition by someone who has a deep appreciation and understanding of the complexities of the gut microbiome.

We've already talked about how the gut and the brain communicate and how the gut can influence many other things that are going on in the body. If you try one and you feel good, then fantastic. But if you try one and you don't feel good, you don't sleep well, you are anxious or something else changes, please do not continue!

While probiotics may help to prevent diarrhoea associated with antibiotic use (94), some concern has been raised in the literature about whether taking probiotics after antibiotic use is the best option for recovering the gut microbiome (95). Mouse models show delays in gut microbiome recovery when probiotics are used (95).

The use and effectiveness here are likely to be highly individual, so this is an area where you should only be taking advice from your (qualified) health practitioner.

Otherwise, you will most likely get a much better result from working on your diet to improve the diversity of the bacteria that you already have there as a base. For most people, this is a much cheaper and safer option.

CHAPTER 27

Fermented Foods?

WATERING YOUR GARDEN

Eating fermented food has been part of human dietary patterns for at least the last 10,000 years. Using bacteria, yeasts and fungi on food helps to stop food spoilage and can in some cases improves taste and textures (96).

Throughout history, foods such as fish, milk, vegetables, beans, cereals and fruits have been specifically prepared to ferment or eaten after natural fermentation has occurred.

Due to the variable nature of fermentation and/or food being fermented, the amount and types of bacterial, yeasts and fungal species present is also highly variable.

I already mentioned previously I wasn't totally sold on the need for probiotics in an isolated pill format because of the complexities of evaluating the evidence here, but fermented foods are a bit different.

There are a huge number of bacterial species present in a fermented food, plus or minus some yeasts and these have become part of the matrix of the food product which was fermented. This makes them much more complex than probiotics, and this is likely to be a good thing in terms of gut health.

The other way that fermented foods might benefit the gut and indeed our overall health is via other bioactive products, produced by the bacteria themselves, as they interact and consume the food they are fermenting.

The complexity of the food matrix and range of species present in fermented food is therefore a good thing!

It is very complicated to measure the impact of different food products on the gut microbiome, because human diets are so complex and there are so many other variables we need to account for in the mix of evaluation. There are also very few studies that have evaluated the actual impact on the gut microbiome using sophisticated techniques such as metagenomic sequencing. What is emerging though, is that fermented foods are good to include as part of our diet. Yoghurt already has a large body of literature supporting its effect on cardiometabolic outcomes and obesity (97,98), but newer research shows that other fermented foods, like sauerkraut, kimchi and kombucha are also associated with increased gut microbiome diversity (99).

I also think it's much easier to include an actual food into your diet than a supplement. It's something that has been around for a long time and you are also getting the added benefits of the nutrients that the fermentation was happening in. For example, yoghurt also contains a good source of protein and calcium, so it has many other benefits beyond the beneficial bacteria.

Yoghurt is an easy one to include as part of your diet, but you could also mix things up now and again and include some sauerkraut or kombucha, knowing they provide many possible benefits, usually without the potential side effects or huge cost of supplements.

CHAPTER 28

You Gut This

WATERING YOUR GARDEN

Some of what you've read here might swirl around in your head for a week or two while you ponder whether you want to make any changes, to work out how to apply some of it to your lifestyle or to work out who you want to show up as in the future. This journey doesn't have to be one that's done in a week or two.

This journey can take a few months or a year or so. What's Important is that you show up for yourself in a small way, consistently. That you feed your gut some good food, that you nurture the aspects of your life that support having a healthier gut, and in return most other things in your life will also start to turn around. Just remember that small changes add up to big ones. You definitely DON'T need to do it all. And you definitely DON'T need to do it all at once.

Now is the time to go and put that list of things you are thankful that your body CAN do on your mirror and stop being mean to yourself about how you look.

I want you to think about something for a minute: How do you want your life to look when you are 80?

The reality is that most people won't achieve that goal of their 80-year-old vision because they don't take enough action NOW to prevent some of the health issues that will inevitably occur in older age without proper strategies in place.

The phrase "use it or lose it" is SO, SO APPLICABLE to the human body. The body does not bother maintaining items that are not used. So, if you don't use your muscles, sorry they're gone. If you don't put stress on your bones with exercise, sorry they're being broken down now too. Science has a much better understanding now that maintenance of muscle mass as we get older could be the single biggest thing we can do to prevent ourselves from so many chronic diseases, from diabetes all the way to dementia. The use of our muscles releases beneficial compounds into the blood stream which can protect our brain and ensure that our pathways for using glucose are efficient.

You will notice that I don't do or provide recipes on my website, this is because well there's a gazillion people already doing that. And let's face it you already know what recipes you like, all you need is a sprinkle of confidence to tweak those recipes and make them a little more gut friendly. Remember you don't need to change everything all at once, you just need to add an extra vegetable or two to start with and this doesn't even need to be part of the recipe, it can be separate on your plate if you like.

So how do we structure our day, our shopping and our plates to make sure we are getting enough gut microbiome food?

Here's a few tips and ideas to give you some inspiration:

- Plan the week's schedule ahead of time (including what you might have for dinner each night)
- Find the recipes you might cook. Have a look at how you can modify them? If you don't want to modify them, then all you need to do is put less of it on your plate and serve yourself up some extra cooked vegetables or salad to go with it.
- Based on the schedule and meals, arrange the groceries you need:

    - If you are making cooked meals, then frozen vegetables are a great option.
    - Pre-cut and washed bags of salad mixes are a great way to increase your vegetable intake without too much hassle. If the budget is tight, then buying a whole lettuce or cabbage as a base is a lot cheaper, so work out what works for you and your budget.
    - Apple cider vinegar, balsamic vinegar or lemon juice are fantastic and cheap dressings to put on your vegetables or salad (also a great low-calorie option).
    - I'm not going to tell you to eat less meat, but it is much cheaper to eat way less of it, and way better for your gut to swap some or all of

the meat, at least a few times per week, with vegetables and legumes.

- What about protein I hear you asking…?? It just so happens that vegetables, breads, pastas and legumes are also good sources of protein. There's some good research around now showing protein suggested intakes for purely avoiding deficiency are not quite optimal for good health, so this is one I also suggest keeping an eye on now and again. If you're getting around 1.2 g/kg of body weight, this is divided throughout the day, then it is likely enough to preserve your muscle mass (86,100,101). Head back to the chapter on protein to make sure you've wrapped your head around this one.
- Fruits, dried fruits and nuts make excellent snacks [if you're worried about the sugars, then pop back to the chapter on fibres, because for most people, these are not a problem]
- Ultra-processed foods can be very cheap and give the illusion of being more cost effective than proper food.

    - I want you to ask yourself though, "Do I feel full after I eat this? Do I even feel good after I eat this?"

- Swapping something ultra-processed, for something higher in fibre will keep you fuller for longer, actually provide food for your gut microbiome and help you get everything else on your list done. There's a choice to be made here!

Aside from these tips, it's a good idea to go back to the table at the start of the book, now that you've digested (pardon the pun) the full meal of information here. Your priorities should be the following:

1. How do you talk to yourself? Make your mind map and your "why" for wanting to be a healthier version of you. Choose yourself and prioritise the work you want to do to get to that better version of you.
2. What is your diet like at the moment? Hold yourself accountable. How much fibre are you eating right now? What foods is it coming from? How much protein, calcium and ultra-processed foods are you eating? What about alcohol? Make a list of all the things you need to or want to improve on.
3. What is your outside time, stress and activity levels like? Be honest with yourself.
4. With this list, choose one SMALL thing to change at a time. This does not have to be diet related, it could be a getting outside goal, a steps goal or something else. The smaller the goal for the

week, the better. **Set yourself up to succeed, not fail**. The goal should be focused on the positive, not anything to do with restriction or negative outcomes.

5. As you make changes, notice how you are feeling. Are you sleeping better, feeling more productive at work? Feeling happier? Your bowel movements better? This can be enough motivation by itself to keep going. Give yourself some thanks and gratitude to your body for responding to your efforts.
6. Find the joy in the process. **This is the most important part**. Sometimes society is so focused on superficial outcomes, we forget to actually stop and have fun. So, stop and admire the shells on the beach or the morning sunshine if you are out and about. Be silly with the kids. Laugh at yourself along the way.

Be the inspiration to yourself. I've written this book because I want you to look back in three to six months and think about all the wonderful changes you made and give yourself a pat on the back. Think about making yourself proud, your kids proud.

Let's create a new generation of people who love and respect their bodies for all the wonderous things it does behind the scenes when no one is watching. A generation of people who care more about being healthy, being fit, being strong and being confident than what we look like.

ABOUT THE AUTHOR

Thank you for choosing to come on a gut centered journey to better health with me. I hope you've learned a few things about yourself and how you want to move forward with your health, starting in the gut.

I really love what I do. This book has actually come to life after a lot of adversity. Most of which involved doing a PhD with three small children in tow, managing a very complex situation at home, and then subsequently navigating life as a single parent. On reflection, all of those hard times have really shaped me and helped me combine my love of science with the kindness and compassion that I think we all need more of these days.

Science is really cool, but the big picture is often lost when new studies make the media or new products get released. The progression of science in this way can fuel those messages about not being enough as we are. I want to change that. The more people that love and appreciate their body for what it CAN do, the more people that will also be able to see the big picture and evaluate the science and the new messages with a bit of critical thinking about whether they need that after all.

Let's spread the message that our body is pretty amazing. If you could actually see all the work it does when we aren't watching, our minds would be seriously blown.

You are awesome. Just as you are. Nurture yourself because you love your body for the right reasons.

If you're interested in one of my programs, my app or just working with me 1:1, please get in contact, I'd love to hear from you. If you enrol in one of my programs, quote promo code BOOK25 for 20% off at checkout.

Otherwise, my email is angela@gutscience.au and the website code is here: https://gutscience.au/

REFERENCES

1. Sun Y, Ju P, Xue T, Ali U, Cui D, Chen J. Alteration of faecal microbiota balance related to long-term deep meditation. Gen Psychiatry. 2023;36(1):e100893.
2. Dulloo AG, Montani JP. Pathways from dieting to weight regain, to obesity and to the metabolic syndrome: an overview. Obes Rev Off J Int Assoc Study Obes. 2015 Feb;16 Suppl 1:1–6.
3. Barber TM, Kabisch S, Pfeiffer AFH, Weickert MO. The Effects of the Mediterranean Diet on Health and Gut Microbiota. Nutrients. 2023 Apr 29;15(9):2150.
4. Pes GM, Dore MP, Tsofliou F, Poulain M. Diet and longevity in the Blue Zones: A set-and-forget issue? Maturitas. 2022 Oct;164:31–7.
5. Parizadeh M, Arrieta MC. The global human gut microbiome: genes, lifestyles, and diet. Trends Mol Med [Internet]. 2023 Oct 1 [cited 2025 Feb 21];29(10):789–801. Available from: https://www.cell.com/trends/molecular-medicine/abstract/S1471-4914(23)00152-1
6. Walter J, Ley R. The Human Gut Microbiome: Ecology and Recent Evolutionary Changes. Annu Rev Microbiol [Internet]. 2011 [cited 2024 Feb

25];65(1):411–29. Available from: https://doi.org/10.1146/annurev-micro-090110-102830
7. Australian Institute of Health and Welfare [Internet]. 2018 [cited 2025 Feb 21]. Australia's health 2018, Fruit and vegetable intake. Available from: https://www.aihw.gov.au/reports/australias-health/australias-health-2018/contents/indicators-of-australias-health/fruit-vegetable-intake
8. David LA, Maurice CF, Carmody RN, Gootenberg DB, Button JE, Wolfe BE, et al. Diet rapidly and reproducibly alters the human gut microbiome. Nature [Internet]. 2014 Jan [cited 2023 Sep 20];505(7484):559–63. Available from: https://www.nature.com/articles/nature12820
9. Takagi T, Naito Y, Inoue R, Kashiwagi S, Uchiyama K, Mizushima K, et al. Differences in gut microbiota associated with age, sex, and stool consistency in healthy Japanese subjects. J Gastroenterol. 2019 Jan;54(1):53–63.
10. Asnicar F, Leeming ER, Dimidi E, Mazidi M, Franks PW, Khatib HA, et al. Blue poo: impact of gut transit time on the gut microbiome using a novel marker. 2021 Sep 1 [cited 2025 Mar 4]; Available from: https://gut.bmj.com/content/70/9/1665
11. Vandeputte D, Falony G, Vieira-Silva S, Tito RY, Joossens M, Raes J. Stool consistency is strongly associated with gut microbiota richness and composition,

enterotypes and bacterial growth rates. Gut. 2016 Jan;65(1):57–62.

12. Appleton J. The Gut-Brain Axis: Influence of Microbiota on Mood and Mental Health. Integr Med Clin J [Internet]. 2018 Aug [cited 2024 Jun 28];17(4):28–32. Available from: https://www.ncbi.nlm.nih.gov/pmc/articles/PMC6469458/
13. Bonaz B, Bazin T, Pellissier S. The Vagus Nerve at the Interface of the Microbiota-Gut-Brain Axis. Front Neurosci [Internet]. 2018 Feb 7 [cited 2024 Aug 15];12. Available from: https://www.frontiersin.org/journals/neuroscience/articles/10.3389/fnins.2018.00049/full
14. Terry N, Margolis KG. Serotonergic Mechanisms Regulating the GI Tract: Experimental Evidence and Therapeutic Relevance. In: Greenwood-Van Meerveld B, editor. Gastrointestinal Pharmacology [Internet]. Cham: Springer International Publishing; 2017 [cited 2025 Feb 21]. p. 319–42. Available from: https://doi.org/10.1007/164_2016_103
15. Loh JS, Mak WQ, Tan LKS, Ng CX, Chan HH, Yeow SH, et al. Microbiota–gut–brain axis and its therapeutic applications in neurodegenerative diseases. Signal Transduct Target Ther [Internet]. 2024 Feb 16 [cited 2024 Aug 15];9(1):1–53. Available from: https://www.nature.com/articles/s41392-024-01743-1

16. Martin CR, Osadchiy V, Kalani A, Mayer EA. The Brain-Gut-Microbiome Axis. Cell Mol Gastroenterol Hepatol [Internet]. 2018 Jan 1 [cited 2024 Aug 15];6(2):133–48. Available from: https://www.sciencedirect.com/science/article/pii/S2352345X18300602
17. Chen CQ, Fichna J, Bashashati M, Li YY, Storr M. Distribution, function and physiological role of melatonin in the lower gut. World J Gastroenterol WJG [Internet]. 2011 Sep 14 [cited 2024 Aug 15];17(34):3888–98. Available from: https://www.ncbi.nlm.nih.gov/pmc/articles/PMC3198018/
18. Iesanu MI, Zahiu CDM, Dogaru IA, Chitimus DM, Pircalabioru GG, Voiculescu SE, et al. Melatonin–Microbiome Two-Sided Interaction in Dysbiosis-Associated Conditions. Antioxidants [Internet]. 2022 Nov [cited 2024 Jun 17];11(11):2244. Available from: https://www.mdpi.com/2076-3921/11/11/2244
19. Yasmin F, Sutradhar S, Das P, Mukherjee S. Gut melatonin: A potent candidate in the diversified journey of melatonin research. Gen Comp Endocrinol [Internet]. 2021 Mar 1 [cited 2024 Aug 15];303:113693. Available from: https://www.sciencedirect.com/science/article/pii/S0016648020304469
20. Akhlaghi M. The role of dietary fibers in regulating appetite, an overview of mechanisms and weight consequences. Crit Rev Food Sci Nutr [Internet]. 2024 Apr 14 [cited 2025 Feb 24];64(10):3139–50.

Available from: https://doi.org/10.1080/10408398.2022.2130160

21. Bodnaruc AM, Prud'homme D, Blanchet R, Giroux I. Nutritional modulation of endogenous glucagon-like peptide-1 secretion: a review. Nutr Metab [Internet]. 2016 Dec 9 [cited 2025 Feb 24];13(1):92. Available from: https://doi.org/10.1186/s12986-016-0153-3
22. Dagbasi A, Byrne C, Blunt D, Serrano-Contreras JI, Becker GF, Blanco JM, et al. Diet shapes the metabolite profile in the intact human ileum, which affects PYY release. Sci Transl Med [Internet]. 2024 Jun 19 [cited 2025 Feb 24];16(752):eadm8132. Available from: https://www.science.org/doi/10.1126/scitranslmed.adm8132
23. Kanchibhotla D, Sharma P, Subramanian S. Improvement in Gastrointestinal Quality of Life Index (GIQLI) following meditation: An open-trial pilot study in India. J Ayurveda Integr Med [Internet]. 2021 Jan 1 [cited 2024 Aug 15];12(1):107–11. Available from: https://www.sciencedirect.com/science/article/pii/S0975947621000085
24. Khine WWT, Voong ML, Ng TKS, Feng L, Rane GA, Kumar AP, et al. Mental awareness improved mild cognitive impairment and modulated gut microbiome. Aging [Internet]. 2020 Dec 9 [cited 2024 Aug 15];12(23):24371–93. Available from: https://www.ncbi.nlm.nih.gov/pmc/articles/PMC7762482/

25. Jimenez MP, DeVille NV, Elliott EG, Schiff JE, Wilt GE, Hart JE, et al. Associations between Nature Exposure and Health: A Review of the Evidence. Int J Environ Res Public Health [Internet]. 2021 Jan [cited 2024 Aug 22];18(9):4790. Available from: https://www.mdpi.com/1660-4601/18/9/4790
26. Buczyłowska D, Zhao T, Singh N, Jurczak A, Siry A, Markevych I. Exposure to greenspace and bluespace and cognitive functioning in children - A systematic review. Environ Res. 2023 Apr 1;222:115340.
27. Nejade RM, Grace D, Bowman LR. What is the impact of nature on human health? A scoping review of the literature. J Glob Health. 2022 Dec 16;12:04099.
28. Song C, Ikei H, Miyazaki Y. Physiological Effects of Nature Therapy: A Review of the Research in Japan. Int J Environ Res Public Health [Internet]. 2016 Aug [cited 2024 Aug 22];13(8):781. Available from: https://www.ncbi.nlm.nih.gov/pmc/articles/PMC4997467/
29. Wen Y, Yan Q, Pan Y, Gu X, Liu Y. Medical empirical research on forest bathing (Shinrin-yoku): a systematic review. Environ Health Prev Med [Internet]. 2019 Dec 1 [cited 2024 Aug 22];24(1):70. Available from: https://doi.org/10.1186/s12199-019-0822-8
30. Zelenski J, Warber S, Robinson JM, Logan AC, Prescott SL. Nature Connection: Providing a Pathway from Personal to Planetary Health.

Challenges [Internet]. 2023 Mar [cited 2024 Aug 22];14(1):16. Available from: https://www.mdpi.com/2078-1547/14/1/16
31. Shin JC, Parab KV, An R, Grigsby-Toussaint DS. Greenspace exposure and sleep: A systematic review. Environ Res. 2020 Mar;182:109081.
32. Raulo A, Allen BE, Troitsky T, Husby A, Firth JA, Coulson T, et al. Social networks strongly predict the gut microbiota of wild mice. ISME J [Internet]. 2021 Sep 1 [cited 2024 Aug 15];15(9):2601–13. Available from: https://doi.org/10.1038/s41396-021-00949-3
33. Pang S, Chen X, Lu Z, Meng L, Huang Y, Yu X, et al. Longevity of centenarians is reflected by the gut microbiome with youth-associated signatures. Nat Aging [Internet]. 2023 Apr [cited 2024 Aug 15];3(4):436–49. Available from: https://www.nature.com/articles/s43587-023-00389-y
34. Dill-McFarland KA, Tang ZZ, Kemis JH, Kerby RL, Chen G, Palloni A, et al. Close social relationships correlate with human gut microbiota composition. Sci Rep. 2019;9(1):703.
35. Johnson KVA. Gut microbiome composition and diversity are related to human personality traits. Hum Microbiome J [Internet]. 2020 Mar 1 [cited 2024 Aug 15];15:100069. Available from: https://www.sciencedirect.com/science/article/pii/S2452231719300181

36. Saeri AK, Cruwys T, Barlow FK, Stronge S, Sibley CG. Social connectedness improves public mental health: Investigating bidirectional relationships in the New Zealand attitudes and values survey. Aust N Z J Psychiatry [Internet]. 2018 Apr 1 [cited 2024 Aug 14];52(4):365–74. Available from: https://doi.org/10.1177/0004867417723990

37. Cai J, Chen Z, Wu W, Lin Q, Liang Y. High animal protein diet and gut microbiota in human health. Crit Rev Food Sci Nutr [Internet]. 2022 Jul 23 [cited 2025 Feb 24];62(22):6225–37. Available from: https://doi.org/10.1080/10408398.2021.1898336

38. Duncan SH, Iyer A, Russell WR. Impact of protein on the composition and metabolism of the human gut microbiota and health. Proc Nutr Soc [Internet]. 2021 May [cited 2025 Feb 24];80(2):173–85. Available from: https://www.cambridge.org/core/journals/proceedings-of-the-nutrition-society/article/impact-of-protein-on-the-composition-and-metabolism-of-the-human-gut-microbiota-and-health/1BB266B926D3A309E9B60B9D4DCDB99E

39. Di Rosa C, Di Francesco L, Spiezia C, Khazrai YM. Effects of Animal and Vegetable Proteins on Gut Microbiota in Subjects with Overweight or Obesity. Nutrients [Internet]. 2023 Jan [cited 2025 Feb 24];15(12):2675. Available from: https://www.mdpi.com/2072-6643/15/12/2675

40. Jenkins DJA, Kendall CWC, Popovich DG, Vidgen E, Mehling CC, Vuksan V, et al. Effect of a very-high-fiber vegetable, fruit, and nut diet on serum lipids and colonic function. Metab - Clin Exp [Internet]. 2001 Apr 1 [cited 2025 Mar 6];50(4):494–503. Available from: https://www.metabolismjournal.com/article/S0026-0495(01)08204-X/fulltext
41. Beasley DE, Koltz AM, Lambert JE, Fierer N, Dunn RR. The Evolution of Stomach Acidity and Its Relevance to the Human Microbiome. PLOS ONE [Internet]. 2015 Jul 29 [cited 2025 Feb 24];10(7):e0134116. Available from: https://journals.plos.org/plosone/article?id=10.1371/journal.pone.0134116
42. Cai J, Rimal B, Jiang C, Chiang JYL, Patterson AD. Bile acid metabolism and signaling, the microbiota, and metabolic disease. Pharmacol Ther [Internet]. 2022 Sep 1 [cited 2025 Feb 24];237:108238. Available from: https://www.sciencedirect.com/science/article/pii/S0163725822001322
43. Liu Y, Zhang S, Zhou W, Hu D, Xu H, Ji G. Secondary Bile Acids and Tumorigenesis in Colorectal Cancer. Front Oncol [Internet]. 2022 Apr 28 [cited 2025 Feb 24];12. Available from: https://www.frontiersin.org/journals/oncology/articles/10.3389/fonc.2022.813745/full
44. Fajstova A, Galanova N, Coufal S, Malkova J, Kostovcik M, Cermakova M, et al. Diet Rich in

Simple Sugars Promotes Pro-Inflammatory Response via Gut Microbiota Alteration and TLR4 Signaling. Cells [Internet]. 2020 Dec 16 [cited 2024 May 16];9(12):2701. Available from: https://www.ncbi.nlm.nih.gov/pmc/articles/PMC7766268/

45. Khan S, Waliullah S, Godfrey V, Khan MAW, Ramachandran RA, Cantarel BL, et al. Dietary simple sugars alter microbial ecology in the gut and promote colitis in mice. Sci Transl Med [Internet]. 2020 Oct 28 [cited 2024 Jun 17];12(567):eaay6218. Available from: https://www.science.org/doi/10.1126/scitranslmed.aay6218
46. Vandeputte D, Joossens M. Effects of Low and High FODMAP Diets on Human Gastrointestinal Microbiota Composition in Adults with Intestinal Diseases: A Systematic Review. Microorganisms [Internet]. 2020 Nov [cited 2025 Feb 24];8(11):1638. Available from: https://www.mdpi.com/2076-2607/8/11/1638
47. Suarez FL, Springfield J, Levitt MD. Identification of gases responsible for the odour of human flatus and evaluation of a device purported to reduce this odour. 1998 Jul 1 [cited 2025 Feb 24]; Available from: https://gut.bmj.com/content/43/1/100.short?casa_token=6WEfq4V4ucIAAAAA:u1Zps083W2H3n-m7qx0gj24PvtINqK5WqRtScXbZRJdKgY2wn-uE-io9ezTC8354_oyZDzOCX-kA

48. Haskey N, Gold SL, Faith JJ, Raman M. To Fiber or Not to Fiber: The Swinging Pendulum of Fiber Supplementation in Patients with Inflammatory Bowel Disease. Nutrients [Internet]. 2023 Jan [cited 2025 Mar 6];15(5):1080. Available from: https://www.mdpi.com/2072-6643/15/5/1080
49. McRorie JW. Evidence-Based Approach to Fiber Supplements and Clinically Meaningful Health Benefits, Part 1: What to Look for and How to Recommend an Effective Fiber Therapy. Nutr Today. 2015 Mar;50(2):82–9.
50. Huwiler VV, Schönenberger KA, Segesser von Brunegg A, Reber E, Mühlebach S, Stanga Z, et al. Prolonged Isolated Soluble Dietary Fibre Supplementation in Overweight and Obese Patients: A Systematic Review with Meta-Analysis of Randomised Controlled Trials. Nutrients [Internet]. 2022 Jan [cited 2024 Dec 16];14(13):2627. Available from: https://www.mdpi.com/2072-6643/14/13/2627
51. Cory H, Passarelli S, Szeto J, Tamez M, Mattei J. The Role of Polyphenols in Human Health and Food Systems: A Mini-Review. Front Nutr [Internet]. 2018 Sep 21 [cited 2024 Jun 18];5:87. Available from: https://www.ncbi.nlm.nih.gov/pmc/articles/PMC6160559/
52. Catalkaya G, Venema K, Lucini L, Rocchetti G, Delmas D, Daglia M, et al. Interaction of dietary polyphenols and gut microbiota: Microbial metabolism

of polyphenols, influence on the gut microbiota, and implications on host health. Food Front [Internet]. 2020 [cited 2023 Sep 5];1(2):109–33. Available from: https://onlinelibrary.wiley.com/doi/abs/10.1002/fft2.25

53. Parmenter BH, Croft KD, Hodgson JM, Dalgaard F, Bondonno CP, Lewis JR, et al. An overview and update on the epidemiology of flavonoid intake and cardiovascular disease risk. Food Funct. 2020 Aug 19;11(8):6777–806.
54. Woodward KA, Draijer R, Thijssen DHJ, Low DA. Polyphenols and Microvascular Function in Humans: A Systematic Review. Curr Pharm Des. 2018;24(2):203–26.
55. Blekkenhorst LC, Bondonno CP, Lewis JR, Devine A, Zhu K, Lim WH, et al. Cruciferous and Allium Vegetable Intakes are Inversely Associated With 15-Year Atherosclerotic Vascular Disease Deaths in Older Adult Women. J Am Heart Assoc [Internet]. 2017 Oct 11 [cited 2025 Mar 6];6(10):e006558. Available from: https://www.ahajournals.org/doi/full/10.1161/JAHA.117.006558
56. Yao ZD, Cao YN, Peng LX, Yan ZY, Zhao G. Coarse Cereals and Legume Grains Exert Beneficial Effects through Their Interaction with Gut Microbiota: A Review. J Agric Food Chem [Internet]. 2021 Jan 27 [cited 2025 Mar 6];69(3):861–77. Available from: https://doi.org/10.1021/acs.jafc.0c05691

57. Farràs M, Martinez-Gili L, Portune K, Arranz S, Frost G, Tondo M, et al. Modulation of the Gut Microbiota by Olive Oil Phenolic Compounds: Implications for Lipid Metabolism, Immune System, and Obesity. Nutrients [Internet]. 2020 Aug [cited 2024 Jun 14];12(8):2200. Available from: https://www.mdpi.com/2072-6643/12/8/2200
58. G. Fraga C, D. Croft K, O. Kennedy D, A. Tomás-Barberán F. The effects of polyphenols and other bioactives on human health. Food Funct [Internet]. 2019 [cited 2025 Feb 24];10(2):514–28. Available from: https://pubs.rsc.org/en/content/articlelanding/2019/fo/c8fo01997e
59. Usuda H, Okamoto T, Wada K. Leaky Gut: Effect of Dietary Fiber and Fats on Microbiome and Intestinal Barrier. Int J Mol Sci [Internet]. 2021 Jan [cited 2025 Feb 14];22(14):7613. Available from: https://www.mdpi.com/1422-0067/22/14/7613
60. John S, Luben R, Shrestha SS, Welch A, Khaw KT, Hart AR. Dietary n-3 polyunsaturated fatty acids and the aetiology of ulcerative colitis: a UK prospective cohort study. Eur J Gastroenterol Hepatol. 2010 May;22(5):602–6.
61. Crimarco A, Landry M, Gardner C. Ultra-processed Foods, Weight Gain, and Co-morbidity Risk. Curr Obes Rep. 2021 Oct 22;11:1–13.
62. Cuevas-Sierra A, Milagro FI, Aranaz P, Martínez JA, Riezu-Boj JI. Gut Microbiota Differences According

to Ultra-Processed Food Consumption in a Spanish Population. Nutrients [Internet]. 2021 Aug [cited 2024 Jun 21];13(8):2710. Available from: https://www.mdpi.com/2072-6643/13/8/2710

63. Hall KD, Ayuketah A, Brychta R, Cai H, Cassimatis T, Chen KY, et al. Ultra-Processed Diets Cause Excess Calorie Intake and Weight Gain: An Inpatient Randomized Controlled Trial of Ad Libitum Food Intake. Cell Metab. 2019 Jul 2;30(1):67-77.e3.
64. Hang D, Du M, Wang L, Wang K, Fang Z, Khandpur N, et al. Ultra-processed food consumption and mortality among patients with stages I–III colorectal cancer: a prospective cohort study. eClinicalMedicine [Internet]. 2024 May 1 [cited 2024 Jun 21];71. Available from: https://www.thelancet.com/journals/eclinm/article/PIIS2589-5370(24)00151-2/fulltext
65. Lane MM, Davis JA, Beattie S, Gómez-Donoso C, Loughman A, O'Neil A, et al. Ultraprocessed food and chronic noncommunicable diseases: A systematic review and meta-analysis of 43 observational studies. Obes Rev [Internet]. 2021 [cited 2024 Jun 21];22(3):e13146. Available from: https://onlinelibrary.wiley.com/doi/abs/10.1111/obr.13146
66. Lane MM, Lotfaliany M, Hodge AM, O'Neil A, Travica N, Jacka FN, et al. High ultra-processed food consumption is associated with elevated psychological distress as an indicator of depression in

adults from the Melbourne Collaborative Cohort Study. J Affect Disord [Internet]. 2023 Aug 15 [cited 2024 Jun 21];335:57–66. Available from: https://www.sciencedirect.com/science/article/pii/S0165032723006092

67. Lane MM, Gamage E, Du S, Ashtree DN, McGuinness AJ, Gauci S, et al. Ultra-processed food exposure and adverse health outcomes: umbrella review of epidemiological meta-analyses. BMJ [Internet]. 2024 Feb 28 [cited 2024 Jun 21];384:e077310. Available from: https://www.bmj.com/content/384/bmj-2023-077310
68. Jian C, Luukkonen P, Sädevirta S, Yki-Järvinen H, Salonen A. Impact of short-term overfeeding of saturated or unsaturated fat or sugars on the gut microbiota in relation to liver fat in obese and overweight adults. Clin Nutr Edinb Scotl. 2021 Jan;40(1):207–16.
69. Song M, Chan AT. Environmental Factors, Gut Microbiota, and Colorectal Cancer Prevention. Clin Gastroenterol Hepatol [Internet]. 2019 Jan 1 [cited 2024 Aug 13];17(2):275–89. Available from: https://www.cghjournal.org/article/S1542-3565(18)30712-2/fulltext
70. Hou CY, Chen YW, Hazeena SH, Tain YL, Hsieh CW, Chen DQ, et al. Cardiovascular risk of dietary trimethylamine oxide precursors and the therapeutic potential of resveratrol and its derivatives. FEBS Open Bio [Internet]. 2024 [cited 2024 Aug 13];14(3):358–

79. Available from: https://onlinelibrary.wiley.com/doi/abs/10.1002/2211-5463.13762

71. Teimouri M, Homayouni-Tabrizi M, Rajabian A, Amiri H, Hosseini H. Anti-inflammatory effects of resveratrol in patients with cardiovascular disease: A systematic review and meta-analysis of randomized controlled trials. Complement Ther Med [Internet]. 2022 Nov 1 [cited 2024 Aug 13];70:102863. Available from: https://www.sciencedirect.com/science/article/pii/S0965229922000656
72. Clauss M, Gérard P, Mosca A, Leclerc M. Interplay Between Exercise and Gut Microbiome in the Context of Human Health and Performance. Front Nutr [Internet]. 2021 Jun 10 [cited 2024 Aug 15];8. Available from: https://www.frontiersin.org/journals/nutrition/articles/10.3389/fnut.2021.637010/full
73. Dalton A, Mermier C, Zuhl M. Exercise influence on the microbiome–gut–brain axis. Gut Microbes [Internet]. 2019 Sep 3 [cited 2024 Aug 15];10(5):555–68. Available from: https://doi.org/10.1080/19490976.2018.1562268
74. Estaki M, Pither J, Baumeister P, Little JP, Gill SK, Ghosh S, et al. Cardiorespiratory fitness as a predictor of intestinal microbial diversity and distinct metagenomic functions. Microbiome [Internet]. 2016 Aug 8 [cited 2024 Aug 15];4(1):42. Available from: https://doi.org/10.1186/s40168-016-0189-7

75. Yang Y, Shi Y, Wiklund P, Tan X, Wu N, Zhang X, et al. The Association between Cardiorespiratory Fitness and Gut Microbiota Composition in Premenopausal Women. Nutrients [Internet]. 2017 Jul 25 [cited 2024 Aug 15];9(8):792. Available from: https://www.ncbi.nlm.nih.gov/pmc/articles/PMC5579588/
76. Zhang YW, Song PR, Wang SC, Liu H, Shi ZM, Su JC. Diets intervene osteoporosis via gut-bone axis. Gut Microbes [Internet]. 2024 Dec 31 [cited 2024 Oct 17];16(1):2295432. Available from: https://doi.org/10.1080/19490976.2023.2295432
77. de Sire A, de Sire R, Curci C, Castiglione F, Wahli W. Role of Dietary Supplements and Probiotics in Modulating Microbiota and Bone Health: The Gut-Bone Axis. Cells. 2022 Feb 21;11(4).
78. Indrio F, Salatto A. Gut Microbiota-Bone Axis. Ann Nutr Metab. 2025 Jan 23;1–10.
79. Tu Y, Yang R, Xu X, Zhou X. The microbiota-gut-bone axis and bone health. J Leukoc Biol. 2021 Sep;110(3):525–37.
80. He Y, Chen Y. The potential mechanism of the microbiota-gut-bone axis in osteoporosis: a review. Osteoporos Int J Establ Result Coop Eur Found Osteoporos Natl Osteoporos Found USA. 2022 Dec;33(12):2495–506.
81. Damani JJ, De Souza MJ, VanEvery HL, Strock NCA, Rogers CJ. The Role of Prunes in Modulating Inflammatory Pathways to Improve Bone Health in

Postmenopausal Women. Adv Nutr [Internet]. 2022 Sep 1 [cited 2024 Nov 10];13(5):1476–92. Available from: https://www.sciencedirect.com/science/article/pii/S2161831323000236

82. Simpson AMR, Souza MJD, Damani J, Rogers C, Williams NI, Weaver C, et al. Prune supplementation for 12 months alters the gut microbiome in postmenopausal women. Food Funct [Internet]. 2022 Nov 28 [cited 2024 Nov 10];13(23):12316–29. Available from: https://pubs.rsc.org/en/content/articlelanding/2022/fo/d2fo02273g
83. Simpson AMR, De Souza MJ, Damani J, Rogers CJ, Williams NI, Weaver CM, et al. Gut microbes differ in postmenopausal women responding to prunes to maintain hip bone mineral density. Front Nutr [Internet]. 2024 Apr 18 [cited 2024 Nov 10];11. Available from: https://www.frontiersin.org/journals/nutrition/articles/10.3389/fnut.2024.1389638/full
84. Key TJ, Papier K, Tong TYN. Plant-based diets and long-term health: findings from the EPIC-Oxford study. Proc Nutr Soc. 2022 May;81(2):190–8.
85. Council NH and MR. Protein [Internet]. 2021 [cited 2025 Mar 7]. Available from: https://www.eatforhealth.gov.au/nutrient-reference-values/nutrients/protein
86. Wolfe RR, Cifelli AM, Kostas G, Kim IY. Optimizing Protein Intake in Adults: Interpretation and Application of the Recommended Dietary Allowance

Compared with the Acceptable Macronutrient Distribution Range. Adv Nutr Bethesda Md. 2017 Mar;8(2):266–75.

87. Simmons E, Fluckey JD, Riechman SE. Cumulative Muscle Protein Synthesis and Protein Intake Requirements. Annu Rev Nutr [Internet]. 2016 Jul 17 [cited 2025 Mar 7];36(Volume 36, 2016):17–43. Available from: https://www.annualreviews.org/content/journals/10.1146/annurev-nutr-071813-105549
88. Abu-Ghazaleh N, Chua WJ, Gopalan V. Intestinal microbiota and its association with colon cancer and red/processed meat consumption. J Gastroenterol Hepatol [Internet]. 2021 [cited 2024 May 16];36(1):75–88. Available from: https://onlinelibrary.wiley.com/doi/abs/10.1111/jgh.15042
89. Kennedy J, Alexander P, Taillie LS, Jaacks LM. Estimated effects of reductions in processed meat consumption and unprocessed red meat consumption on occurrences of type 2 diabetes, cardiovascular disease, colorectal cancer, and mortality in the USA: a microsimulation study. Lancet Planet Health. 2024 Jul;8(7):e441–51.
90. Shi W, Huang X, Schooling CM, Zhao JV. Red meat consumption, cardiovascular diseases, and diabetes: a systematic review and meta-analysis. Eur Heart J. 2023 Jul 21;44(28):2626–35.

91. National Health Council NH and MR. Introduction [Internet]. 2022 [cited 2025 Feb 24]. Available from: https://www.eatforhealth.gov.au/nutrient-reference-values/introduction

92. Medical Research Council NH and MR. Vitamin C [Internet]. 2021 [cited 2025 Feb 11]. Available from: https://www.eatforhealth.gov.au/nutrient-reference-values/nutrients/vitamin-c

93. Vaclavik L, Krynitsky AJ, Rader JI. Mass spectrometric analysis of pharmaceutical adulterants in products labeled as botanical dietary supplements or herbal remedies: a review. Anal Bioanal Chem [Internet]. 2014 Nov 1 [cited 2025 Feb 24];406(27):6767–90. Available from: https://doi.org/10.1007/s00216-014-8159-z

94. Goodman C, Keating G, Georgousopoulou E, Hespe C, Levett K. Probiotics for the prevention of antibiotic-associated diarrhoea: a systematic review and meta-analysis. 2021 Aug 1 [cited 2025 Feb 14]; Available from: https://bmjopen.bmj.com/content/11/8/e043054.abstract

95. Suez J, Zmora N, Zilberman-Schapira G, Mor U, Dori-Bachash M, Bashiardes S, et al. Post-Antibiotic Gut Mucosal Microbiome Reconstitution Is Impaired by Probiotics and Improved by Autologous FMT. Cell [Internet]. 2018 Sep 6 [cited 2025 Feb 14];174(6):1406-1423.e16. Available from: https://www.cell.com/cell/abstract/S0092-8674(18)31108-5

96. Taylor BC, Lejzerowicz F, Poirel M, Shaffer JP, Jiang L, Aksenov A, et al. Consumption of Fermented Foods Is Associated with Systematic Differences in the Gut Microbiome and Metabolome. mSystems [Internet]. 2020 Mar 17 [cited 2025 Feb 15];5(2):10.1128/msystems.00901-19. Available from: https://journals.asm.org/doi/full/10.1128/msystems.00901-19
97. Le Roy CI, Kurilshikov A, Leeming ER, Visconti A, Bowyer RCE, Menni C, et al. Yoghurt consumption is associated with changes in the composition of the human gut microbiome and metabolome. BMC Microbiol [Internet]. 2022 Feb 3 [cited 2025 Feb 18];22(1):39. Available from: https://doi.org/10.1186/s12866-021-02364-2
98. Soedamah-Muthu SS, de Goede J. Dairy Consumption and Cardiometabolic Diseases: Systematic Review and Updated Meta-Analyses of Prospective Cohort Studies. Curr Nutr Rep. 2018 Dec;7(4):171–82.
99. Wastyk HC, Fragiadakis GK, Perelman D, Dahan D, Merrill BD, Yu FB, et al. Gut-microbiota-targeted diets modulate human immune status. Cell. 2021 Aug 5;184(16):4137-4153.e14.
100. Al-Nimr RI. Optimal Protein Intake during Weight Loss Interventions in Older Adults with Obesity. J Nutr Gerontol Geriatr. 2019;38(1):50–68.
101. Yeung SSY, Chan RSM, Woo J. Protein and physical activity in older persons. Curr Opin Clin Nutr Metab Care. 2021 Jan;24(1):42–7.

Made in United States
Orlando, FL
11 May 2026

81383943R00108